17 of the Most Effective Glute Workouts to Grow and Define the Booty At Home

By

S. Cardenas

Table of Contents

Disclaimer

The information provided in this book is correct to the knowledge of the author. Nevertheless, any information you derive from this book should not serve as a substitute to professional medical advice and treatment. After reading this book in its entirety, you, the reader, are encouraged to review related literature.

You are also advised to consult your doctor first to find out if you have any underlying condition that makes it hard for you to improve your buttocks size. Furthermore, you should get proper diagnosis regarding your past or existing injury and health condition. You should seek approval from your doctor before you carry out any of the exercises included in this book. Do not proceed to exercising if he or she disapproves of you doing any exercise, specifically the ones featured in this book, which may adversely affect your health.

This book was written without taking into account your individual physical condition and needs. Therefore, you should not expect the results to be the same among all readers who carry out the exercises included in this book.

The author holds no liability over how you utilize the information provided in this book. You are encouraged to carry out the exercises as safely as you can. Any injury or damage to property resulting from the performance of an exercise featured herein is the sole responsibility of the doer.

Introduction

Thank you for considering this book in your quest for a big booty!

Nowadays having a butt that stands out is among the body goals of women and men alike. This book will further help you understand the appeal behind it. But more importantly, this will introduce you to the healthy and efficient ways of improving your bottom's size.

If you're one of those who aren't blessed with a great behind, this book will fit you perfectly. Featured herein is a list of booty workouts that are all doable and inexpensive. There's no need for you to subscribe to a monthly gym membership, hire a workout trainer, or buy bulky workout equipment. With the exercises included in this book, enhancing your bum can be done in the comfort of your home and with the help of a few gears. And even better, there are pictures provided for each exercise to show you how each workout is done!

While the exercises listed in this book are all for improving your butt, they often come with additional health benefits. Aside from exercises, additional tips are also added to help you achieve your dream bum sooner. Get to know these benefits and tips as you read this book. I made this book to be straight forward and provide you a list of the most effective workouts for the booty that will help you increase its shape. Stay consistent and you will see results.

Thanks again for downloading this book. Have fun reading and exercising!

What Makes Up Your Bum

Before you proceed to any butt-enhancing workout, you need to understand first what makes up your bum. Perhaps, you have encountered the term glutes before. Glutes is an informal term referring to the gluteal muscles which consist of gluteus maximus, gluteus medius and gluteus minimus, with the gluteus maximus as the biggest and nearest to the skin. All in all, these muscles mainly form your buttocks' size and shape. Obviously, training these muscles can boost the overall appearance of your bum.

Aside from the gluteal muscles, your bum is also made up of skin, subcutaneous fat and posterior muscles. Even if you have pimples, cellulites, stretch marks or other skin problems on your behind, these will not influence the shape of your butt. However, your skin may stretch when growing the booty and therefore, might cause stretch marks if you are more prone to them. Having some cocoa butter handy during your journey of growing the booty and continually following these exercises would be helpful in preventing some stretch marks from forming.

The softness of the butt is largely attributed to the layer of fat right beneath the skin, also known as the subcutaneous fat. This type of fat can be found in other parts of the body, but unlike the one in your bum, the presence of this fat elsewhere doesn't seem pleasant at all. This fat is also a health risk when it's located near your internal organs. Unlike your muscles, though, you can't do much regarding the fat in your butt as its distribution and quantity are mainly controlled by your genes and hormones. Thanks to the hormone estrogen, women tend to store more fats in their buttocks region compared to men.

As to the posterior muscles—or the muscles found at the back of your glutes—they can't greatly affect the shape of your butt as they are located relatively far from the skin. Moreover, simply training your glutes can already enhance the firmness and efficiency of the posterior muscles.

Now that you know what mainly determines your butt size, you can understand why exercising your gluteal muscles is an ideal way of improving it. The question now is how to do it easily, safely and effectively.

Glute Workout Basics

Glute workouts are generally safe provided that you adhere to instructions and that you're free from any injury. While you may be doing them solely for improving your bum, you are likely to end up enhancing your overall strength and stamina. Additional benefits include better posture, fat loss and injury prevention.

Due to prolonged sitting, your gluteal muscles become inactive, making them unable to do their basic functions such as providing support when you walk, run, climb or turn. It causes you flat butt as well. The good news is that activating your glutes simply requires working out.

Preparation

Exercising your way to your ideal butt size is possible, but it tends to take time. Nevertheless, there's no need to sacrifice working hours just to accommodate a 30- to 60-minute workout. You can simply allot such time before you prepare for work in the morning or after you arrive in your home in the afternoon or evening.

If you already have a fixed workout routine, preparing for additional exercises for your glutes shouldn't be that hard. Aside from time allotment, finding workout essentials (such as clothes, shoes, mat, and resistance band) won't be much of a challenge. In case you don't have dumbbells or barbell at home, you may want to invest in them though. In addition to glute workouts, you may also use them for enhancing the function and appearance of the others parts of your body. In all honesty, adding weights to glute exercises is the key to what allows your booty to gain a bigger shape and a rounder look.

Committing to a workout feels too hard, though, if you're a newbie who wants to train at home. To help you remain committed, you should design a workout schedule which you are comfortable with. If you want, you can opt to work out for only three days a week. You may start with only a few glute exercises which may only last for around 30 minutes. It will take you more weeks or months to get notable results, but at least you don't feel too burdened by the idea of working out for more days.

You may choose to sustain such schedule until you get to your ideal butt size. Another option is to improve the frequency to five days and/or to increase the number of glute exercises you do in each training session.

As to your workout sessions, they should be consisted of three stages: warming up, training and cooling down. Basically, the warming up stage prepares your body for the training stage which consists of the rigorous glute exercises. The cooling down stage comes last and it's intended to minimize the soreness from the workout and speed up your recovery.

Jogging, skipping and stretching can make up your warming up stage. You may do these for five to 10 minutes. Afterwards, you may proceed to your preferred glute exercises. Lastly, perform breathing and stretching exercises for five to 10 minutes as part of your cooling down stage.

One last note before you start growing your booty: I encourage you to take a picture of your body before starting your journey, specifically the glutes. This will not only help as motivation for you, but also as something to compare to down the road. As you keep performing the exercises, you can refer back to that picture and see the difference in your bum size!

Side Note:

By the way, Some of the workout equipment shown in this book can be found on Amazon.com. Products used in this book are workout bands and dumbbells or Kettlebells. Good quality workout bands can be found for around $10-$15 on Amazon.com. Just make sure to read reviews and compare quality. A good pair of dumbbells ranging from 3lbs-5lbs could cost around $10 as well. Dumbbells can be found online at amazon.com or at Target and other stores. Kettlebells can be found also in store or online. All the weights should be challenging but not unbearably heavy. Start low enough to handle. Its fairly inexpensive to buy these products but they will make quite a difference when it comes to these workouts. So these products are highly recommended.

Do NOT be afraid to lift weights and incorporate the resistance bands or weights in these workouts. These are key to increase size of the glutes. For women, weights will not make you look "bulky" or "manly." This is a misconception. Weights will actually make you look tone and leaner. So ladies, do not be afraid to lift those weights.

Stretching Exercises

Stretching exercises may or may not have an impact on your gluteal muscles. However, they help prepare your body for workout and minimize the soreness afterwards, so it's important for you to know how to do them properly. Another benefit of stretching is that it improves your flexibility and relieves tensed muscles. Below are stretching exercises you can do for specific body parts.

For Sides of Neck:

1. Stand or sit with your hands on your waist or with your arms hanging loosely on your sides.
2. Turn your head to one side for five seconds, then to other side for another five seconds.
3. Repeat step 2 for three times.
4. Relax.
5. Next, tilt your head to one side for five seconds, then to other side for another five seconds.
6. Repeat step 5 for three times.
7. Relax.

For Back of Neck:

1. Stand or sit with your hands on your waist or with your arms hanging loosely on your sides.
2. Slowly tilt your head forward. Hold it for five seconds.
3. Straighten your neck for a second.
4. Slowly tilt your head backwards. Hold it for five seconds.
5. Repeat steps 2 to 4 for three times.
6. Relax.

For Back of Upper Arms and Sides of Shoulders:

1. Stand or sit with your right hand on your left shoulder.
2. Using your left hand, pull your right elbow towards your left shoulder. Hold it for 10 to 15 seconds.

3. Repeat step 2 on the other side.
4. Relax.

For Back, Shoulders, Arms, Wrists and Fingers:

1. Clasp your hands.
2. Turn your palms out.
3. Extend your arms overhead. Hold it for 10 to 15 seconds.
4. Repeat one more time.
5. Relax.
6. Clasp your hands behind you.
7. Turn your palms out.
8. Extend your arms upward. (It's okay if you can only extend them at waist level.) Hold it for 10 to 15 seconds.
9. Repeat one more time.
10. Relax.

For Top of Shoulders, Triceps and Waist:

1. Stand with your knees slightly bent.
2. Raise your arms overhead.
3. Using your left hand, hold the elbow of your right arm.
4. Gently pull the elbow towards the back of your head.
5. Slowly lean to your right side. Maintain the position for 10 to 15 seconds.
6. Repeat the steps on your left arm.
7. Relax.

For Middle Back:

1. Stand with your hands on your hips, your knees slightly bent and your feet shoulder-width apart.
2. Gently twist your upper body to one side. Hold it for 10 to 15 seconds.
3. Repeat on the other side.
4. Relax.

For Calves:

1. Stand facing a wall and with your arms on your sides.
2. Raise your right forearm and rest your head on it. Slowly lean on the wall with your forearm serving as a cushion.
3. Put your right foot forward, bending your right leg. Keep your left leg straight behind. Hold it for 10 to 15 seconds.
4. Repeat on the other side.
5. Relax.

For Front of Thighs:

1. Stand with your left hand on a wall for support.
2. Using your right hand, grab your right foot without bending your upper body or left leg.
3. Pull your right heel towards your butt. Hold it for 10 to 15 seconds.
4. Repeat on the other side.
5. Relax.

For Calves, Hamstrings and Ankles:

1. Stand with your feet shoulder-width apart.
2. Slightly bend your knees. (It's a bit similar to squat position but your thighs don't have to be parallel to the floor.) Hold the position for 30 to 60 seconds.
3. Relax.

For Inner Thighs and Groin:

1. Stand with your hands on your hips and your feet around 20 inches apart (or wider).
2. Slowly bend your right knee, moving your left hip downward. Put your weight on your right foot. Hold the position for 10 to 15 seconds.
3. Repeat on your left knee.
4. Relax.

For Hips and Hamstrings:

1. Sit on the floor (or on your workout mat) with your legs straight out in front.
2. Bend your left leg and place your left foot outside your right knee.
3. Using both your hands, pull your left knee towards you right shoulder. Hold it for 10 to 15 seconds.
4. Repeat on the other side.
5. Relax.

For Neck, Hips and Lower Back:

1. Sit on the floor (or on your workout mat) with your legs straight out in front.
2. Bend your left leg and place your left foot outside your right knee.
3. Bend your right elbow and rest it on your left knee.
4. Put your left hand on the floor behind you.
5. Turn your head over your left shoulder. Hold the position for 10 to 15 seconds.
6. Repeat on the other side.
7. Relax.

For Lower Back and Back of Leg:

1. Sit on the floor (or on your workout mat) with your legs spread out.
2. Bend your right knee with your leg and ankle resting on the floor or mat.
3. Slowly bend your hips forward until you feel stretched. Hold it for 10 to 15 seconds.
4. Repeat on the other side.
5. Relax.

For Ankles:

1. Stand with your feet shoulder-width apart. Grab or lean onto something for balance.

2. Raise your right foot and rotate it clockwise for 10 times. Rotate it counterclockwise for 10 times.
3. Repeat on your left foot.
4. Relax.

For Shoulders, Arms and Feet:

1. Lie on your back. Keep your back and legs straight.
2. Extend your arms overhead.
3. Stretch for five seconds.
4. Relax.

Stretching exercises are light in nature so it's safe to do them every day. Just don't overexert when you have an injury. You can do them right after you wake up to shake off your sleepiness. You may also do some stretching in the office to ease and prevent muscle tension. As to your glute exercises, do as many stretching exercises as you can. You may lessen the reps to speed up your warm up and cool down stages.

List of Glute Exercises

It is almost time to start exercising! Just keep in mind, the exercises discussed below are to target the glutes and may help with other muscle areas. So if you are ready to start growing a booty, keep reading.

What makes a workout more effective for improving your glutes is the use of weights (whether it's dumbbells, barbell or kettlebell) and your own body weight. While weights make exercising more strenuous, you can actually get more rewards which include bigger bum and stronger thighs. They may speed up the process for you as well. Below are the glute workouts you can include in your training sessions at home. Start the workouts about 2-3 times week and see the results!

Squat (3 sets of 10 reps)

Squats are basic components of workout routines. They are mainly designed to enhance your strength but hey can also boost your booty size provided that you do them properly. Before you do squats (or any other glute exercise for that matter), make sure you get rid of excess fats first. But if your bum is flat due to inactive glutes, squatting can help activate and harden them.

Squats are generally easy. However, poor posture and improper workout clothes can make them a bit harder and even increase the risk of injury.

Instructions:

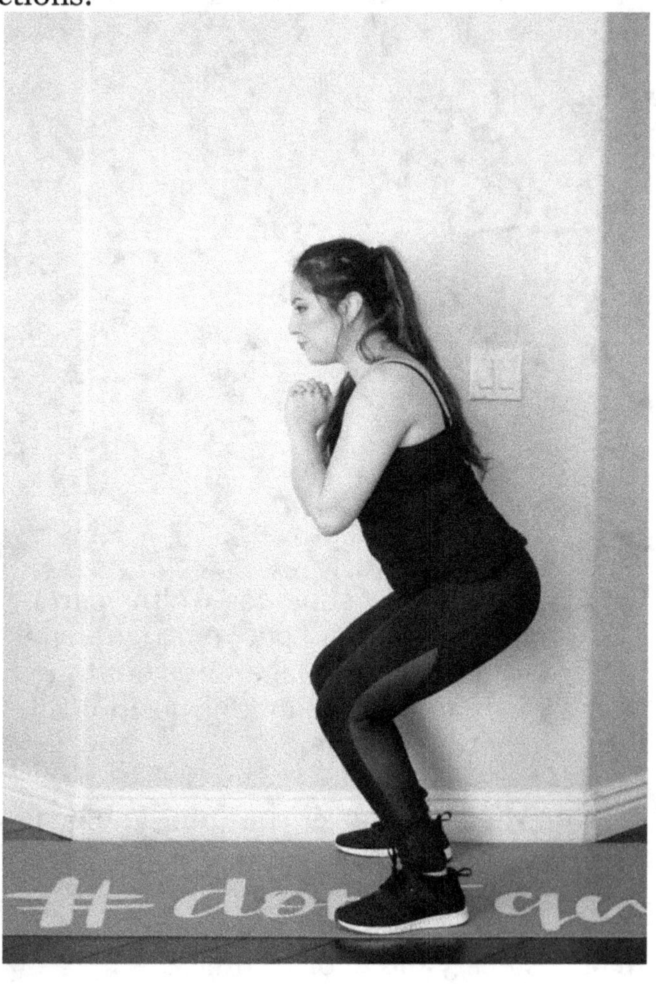

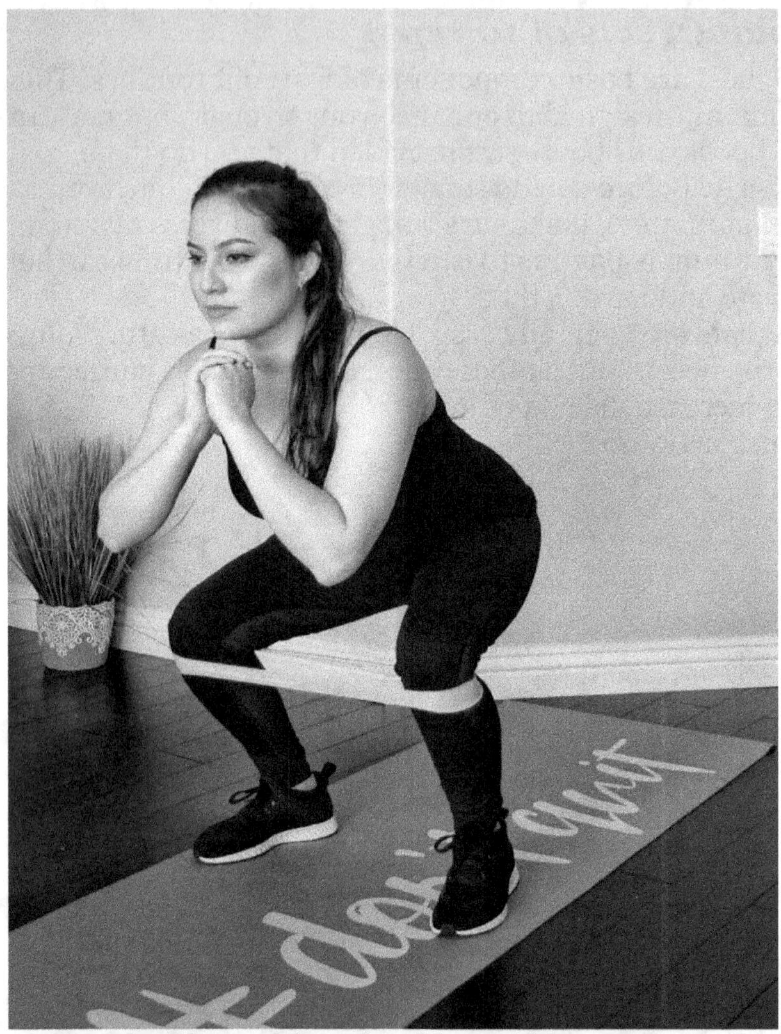

1. Stand with your feet shoulder-width apart.
2. Close your left hand and put your right hand over it. Bend your elbows and make sure your thumbs are facing your chest. Maintain this position all throughout the exercise.

3. Tighten your core, lower your hips and bend your knees until they are parallel to the floor. Hold this position for 10 to 15 seconds.
4. Straighten your legs for five seconds.
5. Repeat steps 3 and 4 for 10 times.

6. After finishing a set of 10 reps, rest for a minute.
7. Do two more sets of 10 reps before resting.

Tips:

- Perform the exercise with a barbell. To do this, skip step 2 and lift the barbell instead. To properly lift a barbell, you should follow the instructions below:
  1. Make sure your feet are straight and shoulder-width apart. Your knees should be pointing out as well.
  2. Bend your hips.
  3. Grab the barbell using both hands. Your hands should be positioned outside your knees.
  4. Next, deadlift the barbell up to your chest.
  5. Afterwards, lift your barbell overhead and place it on your back. Make use of a barbell pad if you find it too painful to carry the barbell this way.
  6. Keep your back straight all throughout and proceed to steps 3 and so on.
- Instead of a barbell, you can also do squats while carrying a kettlebell. This also requires skipping step 2. Below is a guideline on how to lift a kettlebell properly.
  1. Hold the handle of the kettlebell using both hands.
  2. Bend your elbows and make sure the kettlebell is on the same level as your chest.
  3. Maintain this position as you proceed to the steps 3 and so on.

Remember: Adding weights to these workouts is key to increasing booty size. As long as you are not straining or working through an injury, adding a barbell, kettlebell or dumbbells are highly recommended.

Squat Jump (3 sets of 10 reps)

Squat jumps take the basic squats to a whole new level of difficulty. But as the difficulty increases, the benefits you can reap also increase. Aside from conditioning your glutes, this squat variation also helps tone your calves and boost the height of your jumps. Before trying out this exercise, make sure your master the basic squats first. You should also practice jumping and landing properly.

Instructions:

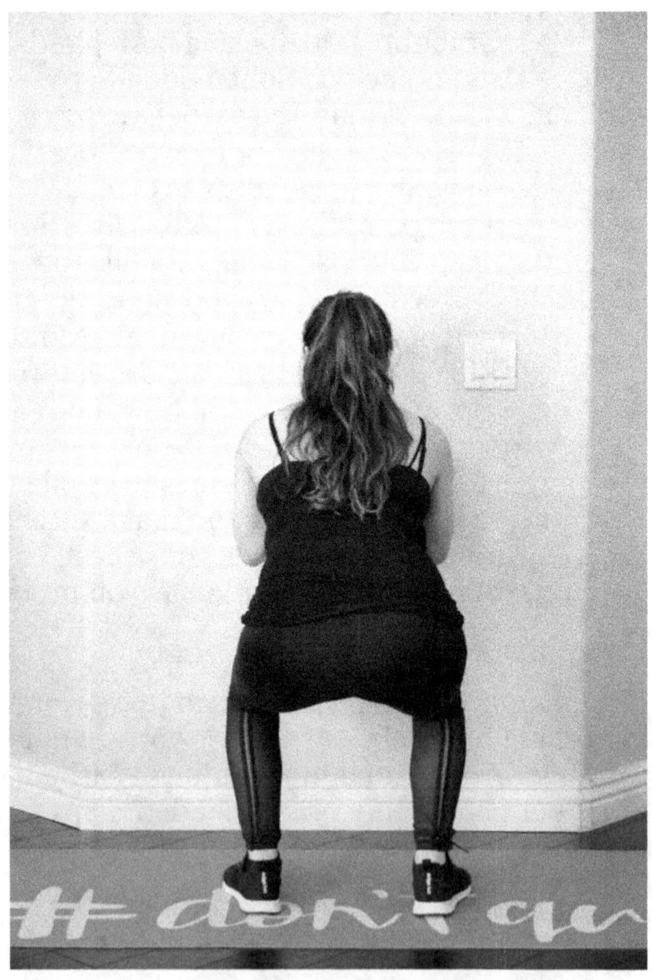

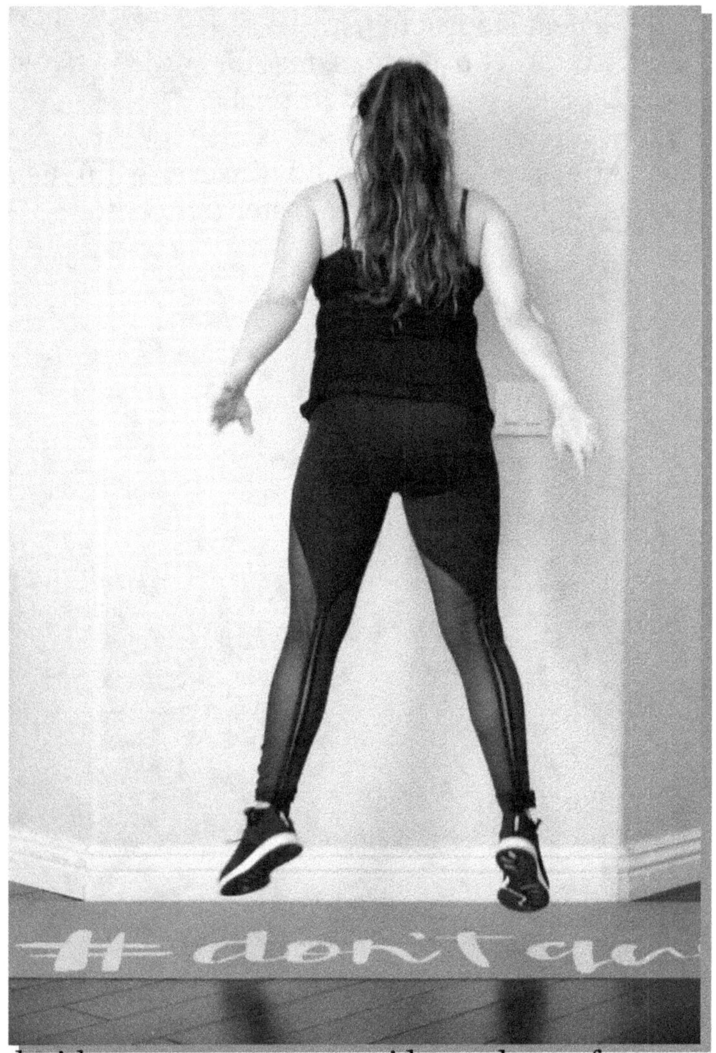

1. Stand with your arms on your sides and your feet shoulder-width apart.
2. Bend your knees until your thighs are parallel to the floor. You can close one hand and cover it with the other hand like in squat position. Keep your back straight.
3. Jump with your arms swinging down by your side.
4. Land softly, put your arms on your sides and return to squat position.
5. Rest for a second or two.

6. Repeat steps 3 to 5 for 10 times.
7. After a set of 10 reps, rest for three to five minutes.
8. Do two more sets of 10 reps.

Tips:

- After perfecting the above exercise, intensify the challenge by jumping faster than before.

Step Up (2 sets of 12 reps per leg)

The step up exercise forces you to carry your body weight against gravity. The benefits you can reap from this exercise are almost similar to the ones you can get from frequently climbing stairs. One of the said benefits is toning your upper hamstrings and glutes.

What You'll Need:

- a sturdy chair or step stool

Instructions:

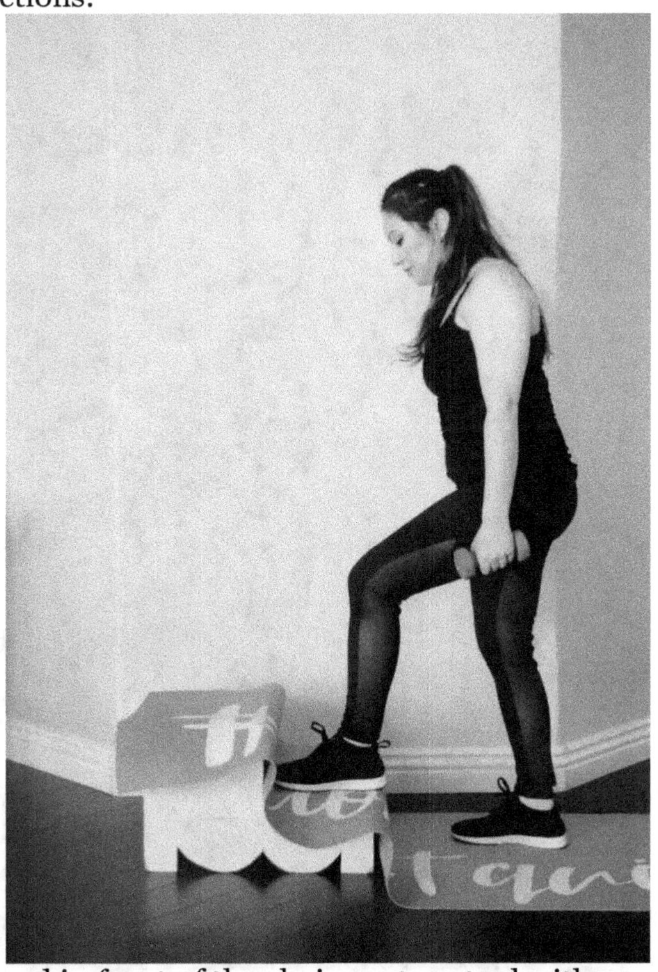

1. Stand in front of the chair or step stool with your fists closed and your elbows bent, making your arms parallel to the floor. Keep your upper body straight (except your arms) all throughout the exercise.

2. Place your right foot on the middle part of the chair or step stool. Swing your right arm backwards as you step up.
3. Transfer your weight on your right heel. Straighten your right leg, causing you to raise your left leg. Make sure your left foot is pointing downwards as you raise your left leg.

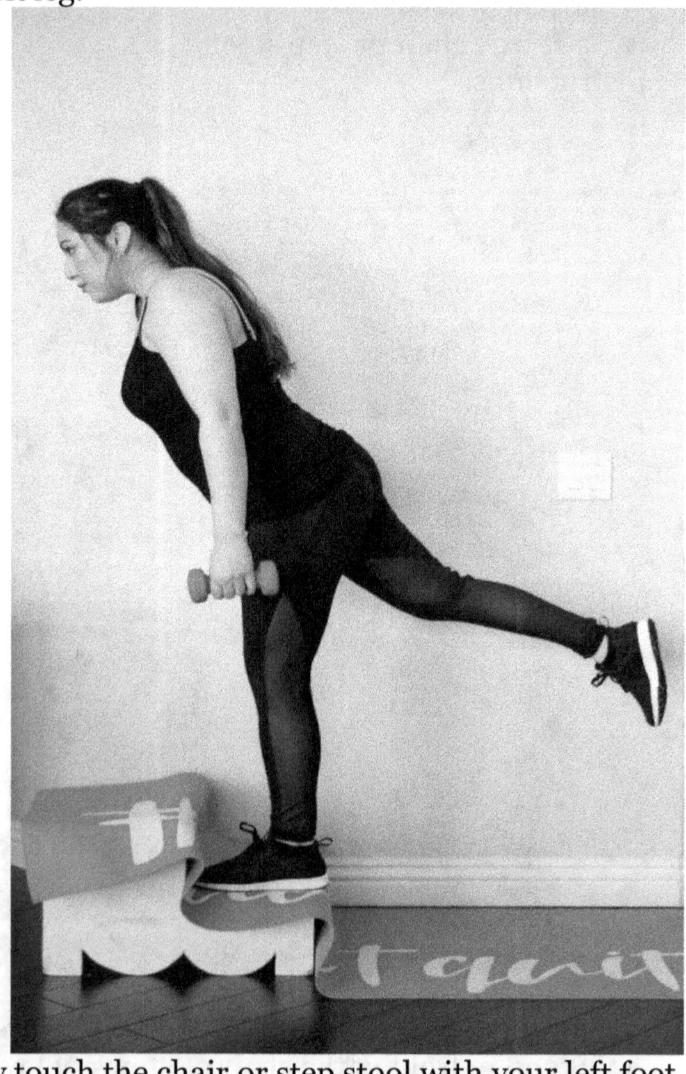

4. Lightly touch the chair or step stool with your left foot pointing downwards

5. Stand on the step with your right leg straight and left leg slightly bent. Hold this position for a second.
6. Bend your right knee, bringing your left foot back to the floor. Keep your left foot on the floor for a second.
7. Repeat steps 3 to 6 for 12 times.
8. After completing a set of 12 reps, perform the exercise with your weight on your left leg.
9. Do a set of 12 reps on your left leg as well.
10. Repeat another set of 12 reps for your right leg and an additional set for your left leg.

Tips:
- Start with a low step. Increase the height as you master a certain height.
- Hold dumbbells as you carry out the exercise. Instead of bending your elbows, put your hands on your sides all throughout the exercise.
- You can increase the challenge by kicking your left (or right) leg as you step up.
- You may also carry out this exercise on a curb or on a stair.

Walking Lunge (2 sets of 12 reps)

Lunges are a favorite exercise of beginners and veterans alike due to their simplicity and efficiency. It has various types; one of which is the walking lunge. Although it's easy to do, this basic lunge helps stretch your hip flexors, making them ideal as additional warming up or cooling down exercise. Plus, they improved the looks and strength of your quads, hamstrings and glutes.

What You'll Need:

- workout mat (recommended)

Instructions:

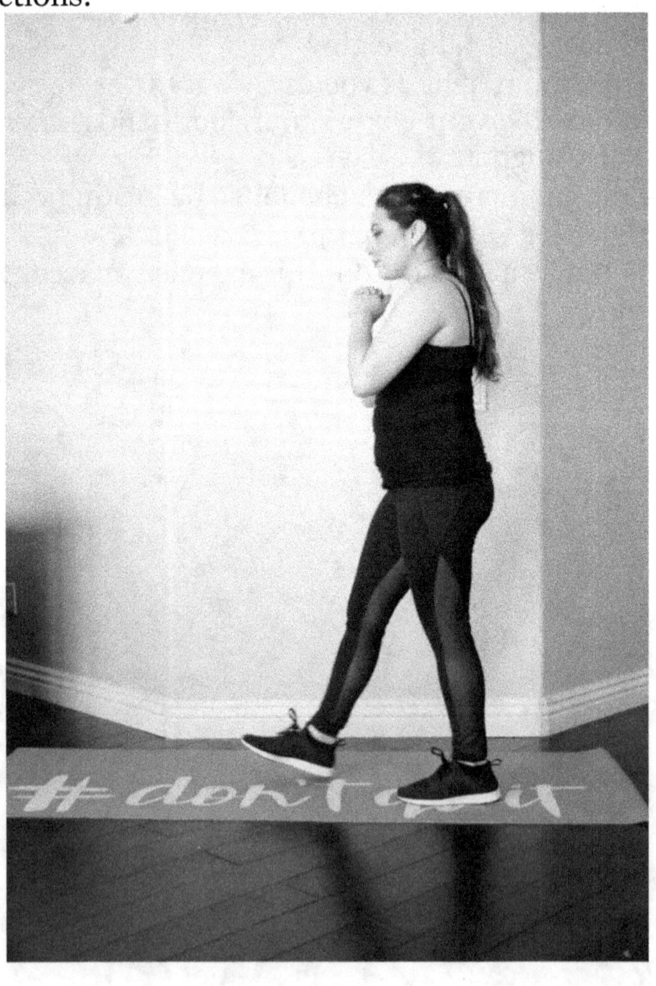

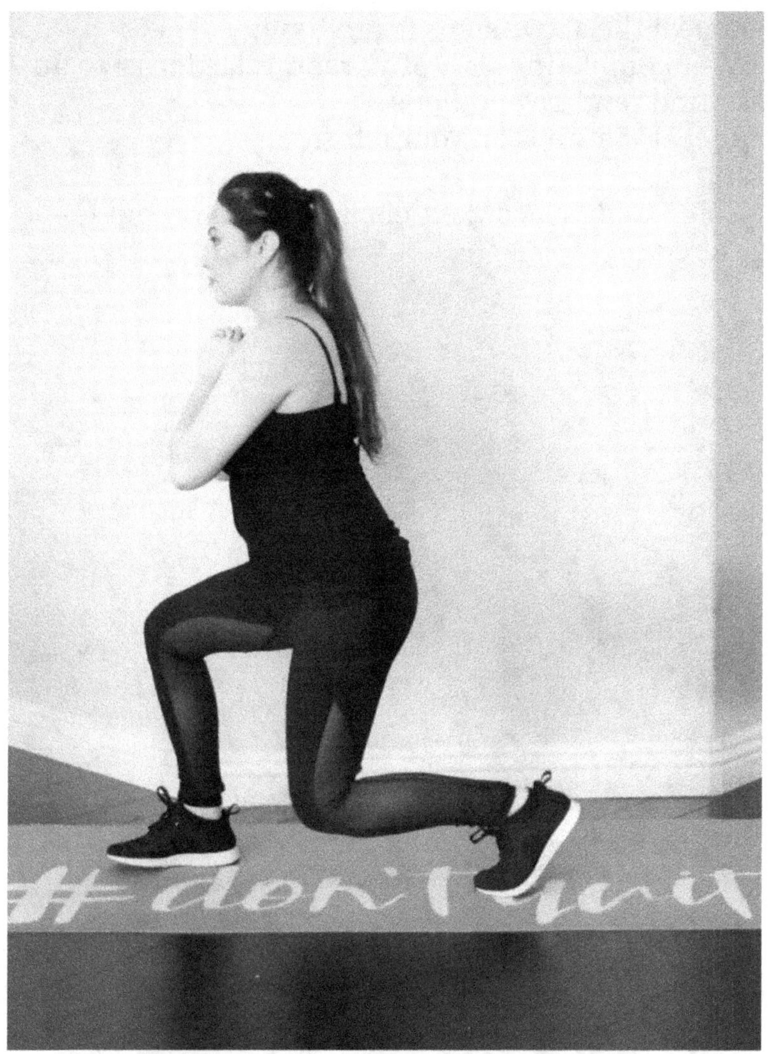

1. Stand with your feet hip-width apart.
2. Using your right leg, step forward and lower your hips.
3. Bend your knees up to an angle of 90 degrees. Your left knee should be pointing downwards but not touching the floor.
4. Put your weight on your right heel and straighten your right leg.
5. Step forward with your left foot, putting you back to starting position.

6. Repeat the above steps for 12 times.
7. After completing a set of 12 reps, relax for 10 to 20 seconds and do another set.
8. Repeat the steps on your left side.

Tips:

*   Hold dumbbells or kettlebell as you carry out the exercise.

Curtsy Lunge (3 sets of 12 reps per leg)

Curtsy lunge engages your gluteus medius and inner thighs. Toned thighs help make your bum appear perkier. In addition to enhancing and strengthening your butt, this variation of the basic lunge also stabilizes your hips and overall posture.

This lunge is also more difficult than the walking, front and reverse lunges because it involves a cross-body movement. Thanks to the cross-body move, though, more muscles in your lower body are used and activated.

Instructions:

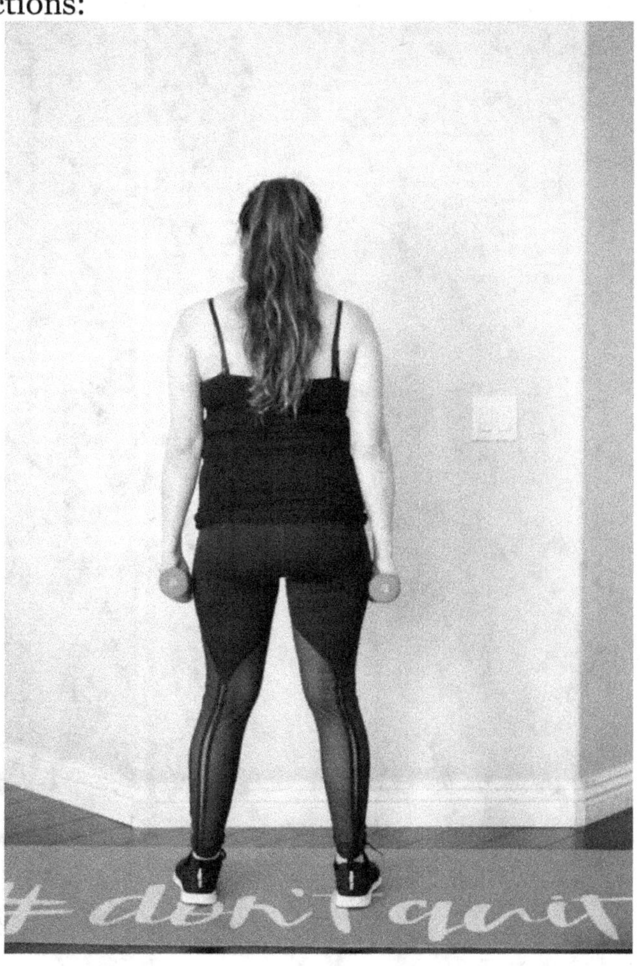

1. Stand straight. Close your left hand and put your right hand above it. Keep your hands this way all throughout the exercise.
2. Bend your elbows. Make sure your hands are in front of your chest.
3. Using your left leg, take a step backwards, towards your right. Step as far as you can.

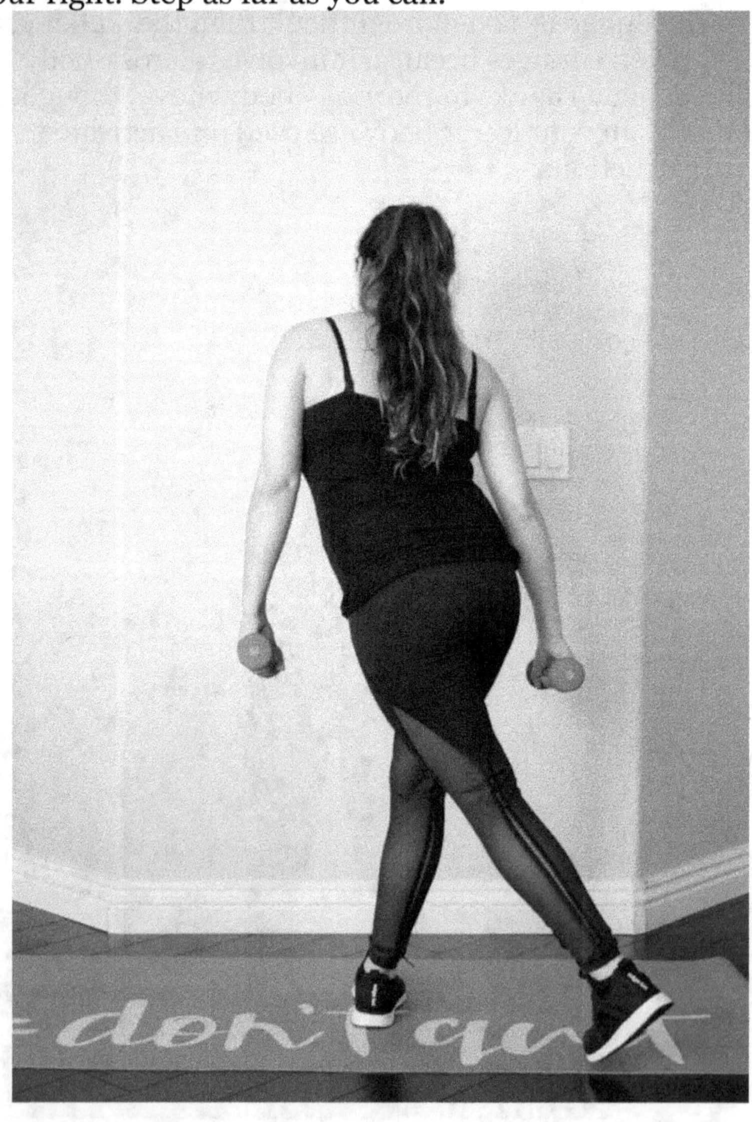

4. As your thighs are crossed, bend both knees. Your right thigh should be parallel to the floor and your

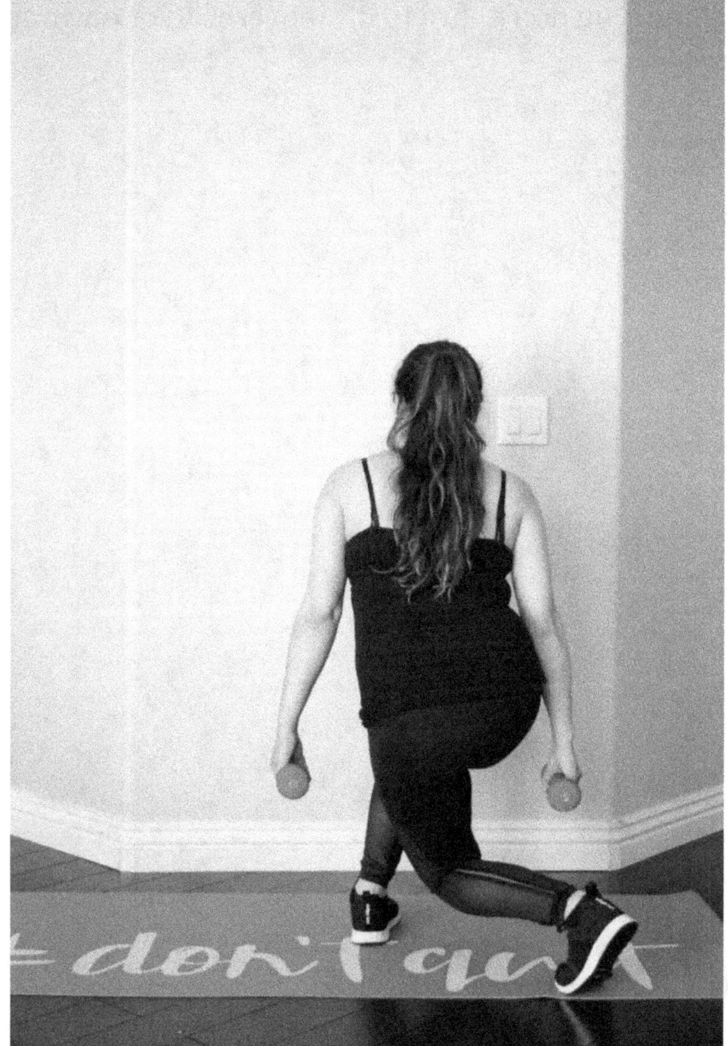

right knee should be aligned with your ankle.
5. Straighten both knees and go back to starting position.
6. Repeat the steps for 12 times.
7. After completing a set of 12 reps, rest for a bit before completing two more sets of 12 reps.
8. Repeat the steps on your other side.

Tips:
- Perform this exercise while lifting a barbell up to your shins. You don't have to lift it overhead or on your back.

Single Leg Deadlift (3 sets of 8 reps per leg)

The single leg deadlift (SLDL) is mainly intended to enhance your overall strength, body coordination and balance. But as you do this exercise, you also end up tightening your glutes.

Deadlifting with both of your feet firmly planted on the ground seems easier and less painful doing it while raising one leg. However, SLDL is proven to be less straining on your back and knees. It activates your glutes faster as well.

What You'll Need:

- barbell or dumbbells (enough weight to challenge but not to injure)

Instructions:

With barbell

1. Stand with your feet shoulder-width apart and in front of your barbell.
2. Shift your weight to your right heel.
3. Raise your left leg backwards, prompting your upper body to lower down.
4. As your upper body becomes almost parallel to the floor, grab the barbell with your hands a little more than shoulder-width apart.
5. Lift the barbell up to the level of your middle or upper shins. Your upper body down to your left leg should be straight while you may slightly bend your right knee. Hold this position for three to five seconds.
6. Slowly lower the barbell down. Return to original position.
7. Repeat steps 3 to 6 for 8 times.
8. After completing a set of 8 reps, rest for a minute or two.
9. Finish two more sets of eight reps.
10. Repeat the steps on your other leg.

With dumbbells

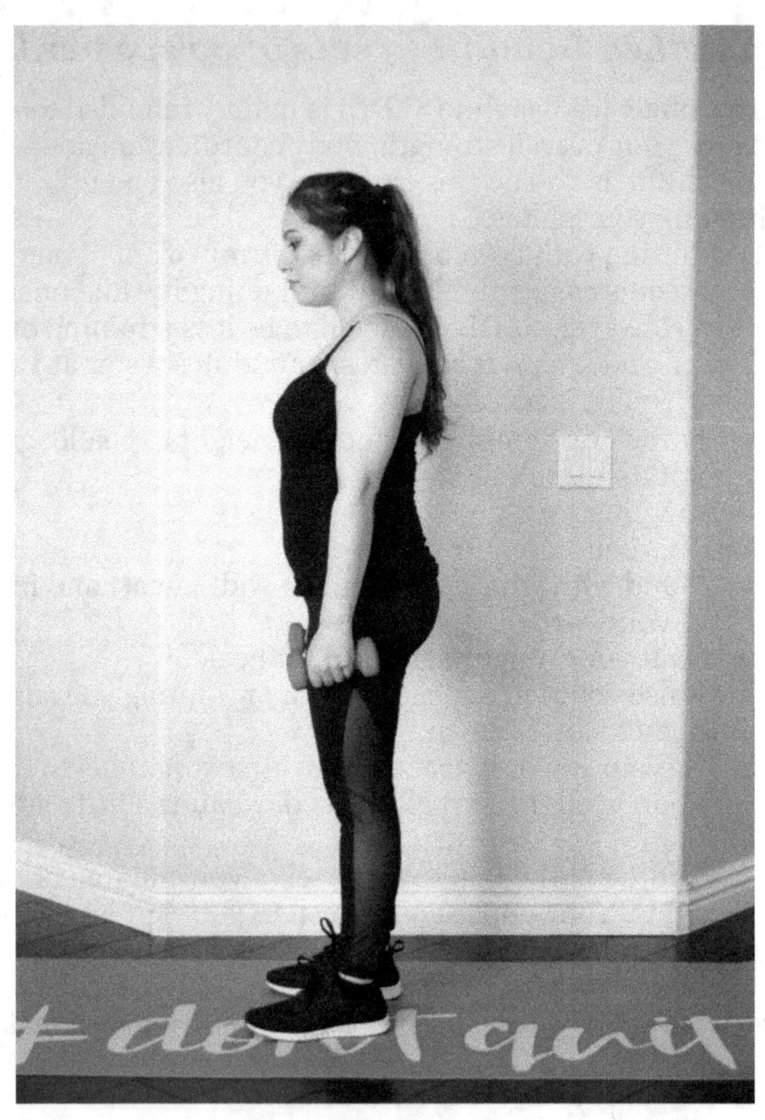

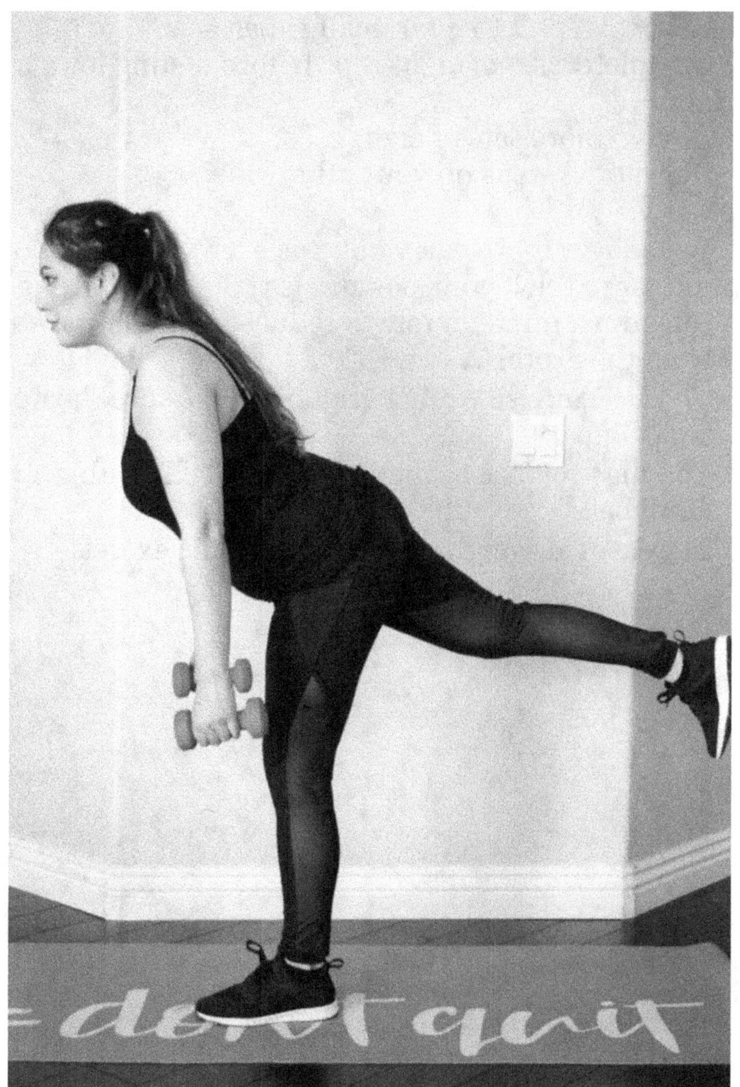

1. Stand with your feet shoulder-width apart. Hold a dumbbell on each hand.
2. Put your weight on your right foot.
3. Raise your left leg backwards, causing your upper body to become almost parallel to the floor (except your arms). Keep your left leg straight while you may slightly bend your right leg. Hold this position for three to five seconds.
4. Lower your left leg and return to original position.

5. Repeat steps 2 to 4 for eight times.
6. Complete a set of eight reps before resting for a minute.
7. Do two more sets of eight reps.
8. Repeat the steps on your other side.

Tips:

- You may want to carry out this exercise in front of a mirror to see if your posture is right. If it's wrong, you can adjust immediately to reduce the potential strain from the exercise.
- Try the exercise while barefoot. Make sure the floor isn't slippery.
- You may replace barbell and dumbbells with a kettlebell.
- Increase the weight as you master the exercise.

Glute Bridge (2 sets of 20 reps)

Glute bridge is one of the fundamental butt-enhancing exercises as it encourages you to squeeze your gluteal muscles. By doing so, it activates, tones and toughens the said muscles. For many women, another benefit of this exercise is that it boosts mind-muscle connection. It also offers great relief for those who are frequently sitting due to the nature of their work or poor lifestyle choices.

What You'll Need:

- workout mat (recommended)
- a form of head support (such as a folded towel)

Instructions:

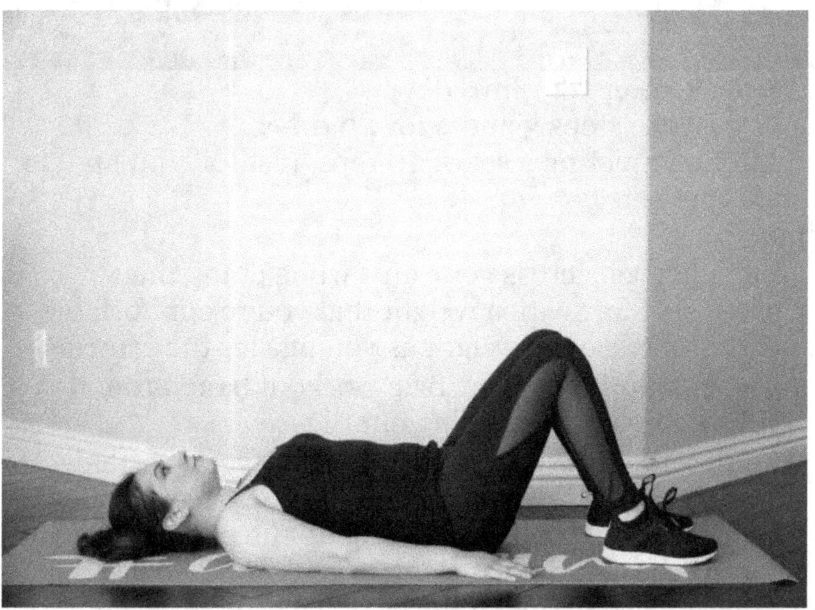

1. Lie on your back with your arms on your sides and palms on the mat. (You may also close your fists, bend your arms and rest your elbows on the mat.) Bend your knees but keep your feet firmly planted on the mat.
2. Squeeze your glutes as hardly as you can.
3. Raise your hips until your knees, hips and shoulders form a straight line. Hold this position for two seconds.

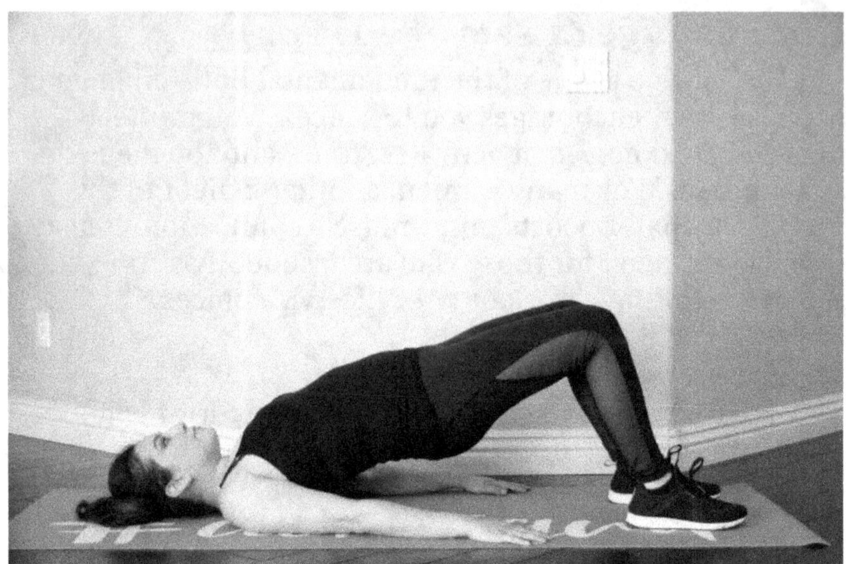

4. Slowly lower your hips down.
5. Repeat the steps 3 and 4 for 20 times.
6. After completing a set of 20 reps, rest for a bit and do another set.

Tips:
- Lift a barbell across your hips while doing this exercise. Start with a weight that you're comfortable with. Increase the weight as you master the exercise.
- Another option is wearing a workout band around your knees while carrying out the exercise.
- Modify the workout by putting your feet on a chair, a step stool or a low table. Elevating your feet further squeezes your glutes, speeding up the process of toning those muscles.
- You can also intensify the exercise by turning your body sideways after your raise your hips.

Single Leg Glute Bridge (2 sets of 20 reps per leg)

The basic difference between the standard glute bridge and single leg glute bridge is that you don't raise one leg in the former. The one-legged glute bridge is slightly harder, but once you master this variation, trying out the more advanced types of glute bridges becomes easier. In addition your butt size, this variation also boosts your running and jumping abilities. Compared to the standard type, this strengthens your core faster.

What You'll Need:

- workout mat (recommended)

Instructions:

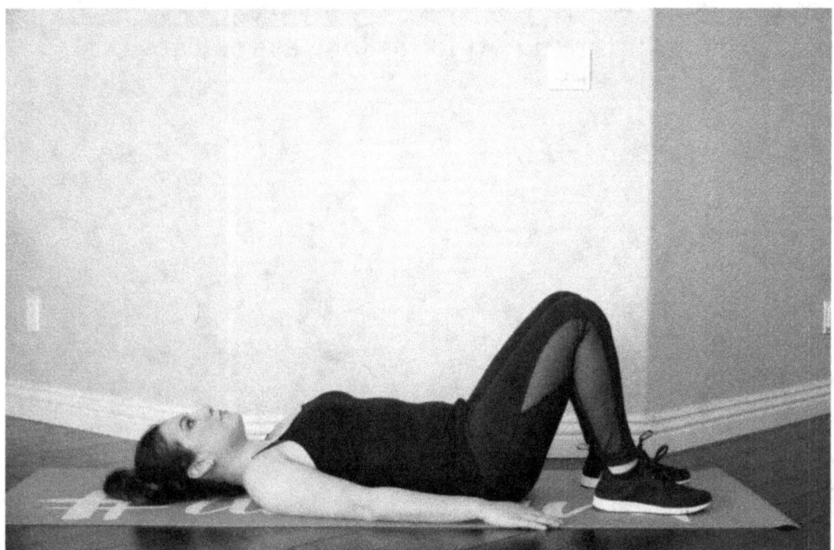

1. Lie on your back with your feet flat on your workout mat and shoulder-width apart. Close your fists, bend your arms and rest your elbows on the mat.
2. Bend your knees.
3. Raise your right foot off the mat and straighten your right leg.

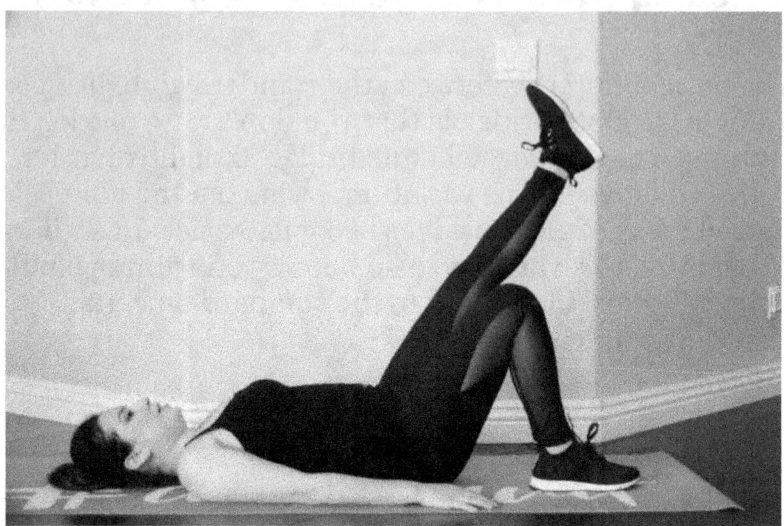

4. Lift your hips and butt for as long as you can.

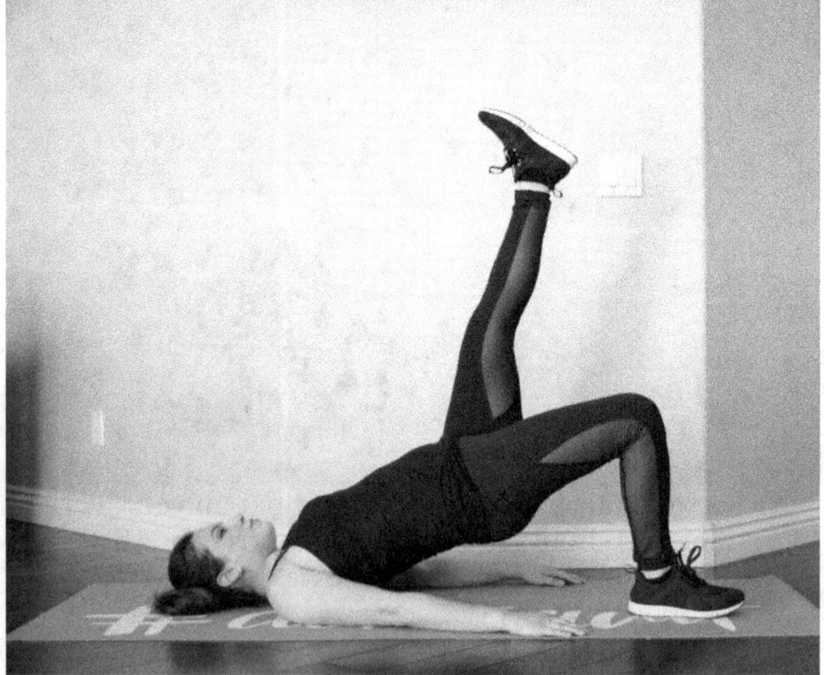

5. Lower your back down but keep your right leg
    straight.
6. Repeat steps 3 to 5 for 20 times.

7. After completing a set of 20 reps, rest for a bit and do another set.
8. Repeat the steps on your other leg.

Tips:

- Make use of a barbell. Lift it across your hips.
- Pull your feet closer to your butt if your hamstrings begin to cramp.
- As you raise one leg, make sure your hips are even.

Fire hydrants (2 sets of 20 reps per leg)

The kneeling hip abduction, better known as fire hydrant, is designed as a lower body exercise but it benefits your hips and abdominal muscles as well. As a glute exercise, fire hydrant tones and strengthens the superficial muscles in your butt and thighs. It also helps you shed fats on your thighs. With slender thighs, your butt is more pronounced. To reap the benefits sooner, make sure your movements are controlled all throughout the exercise.

Fire hydrants are best done at the beginning of your training session. You may follow it up with donkey kicks or squats.

What You'll Need:

- workout mat (recommended)

Instructions:

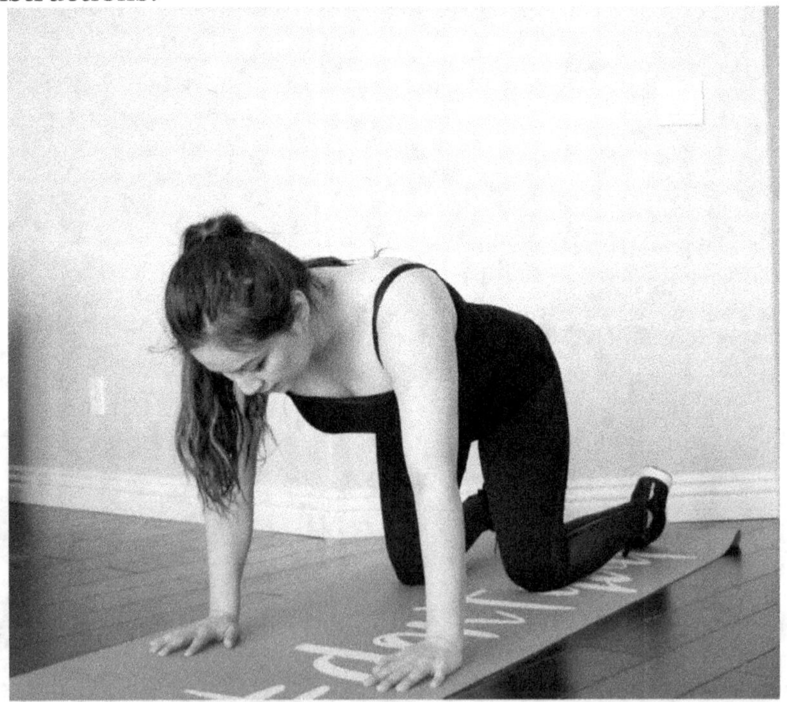

1. Go down on all fours with your palms flat to the mat and shoulder-width apart while your feet are hip-width apart.
2. Bend your knees to an angle of 90 degrees. Make sure your back is straight all throughout the exercise.

3. Raise your left thigh close to your chest.

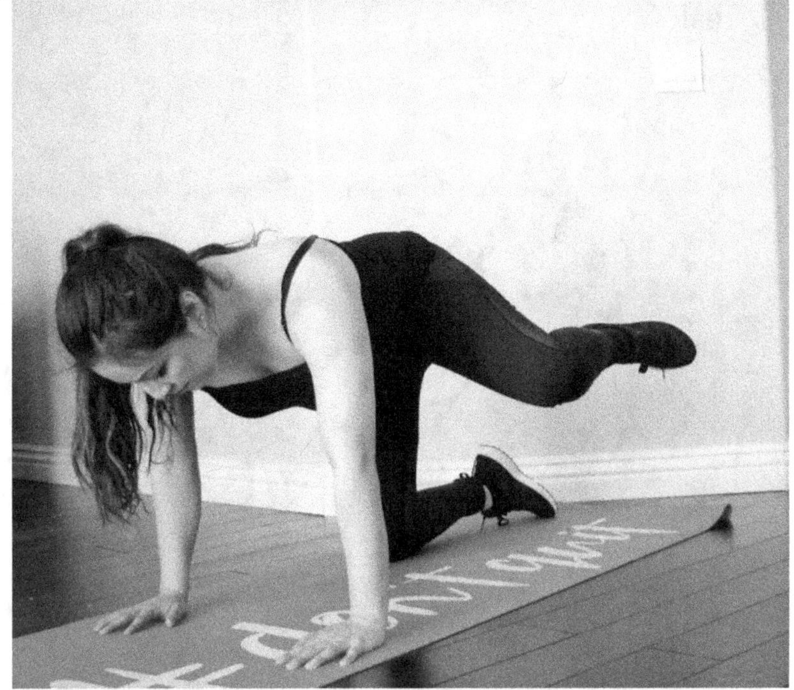

4. Raise the said thigh to your side without moving your hips. Hold it for a second.
5. Slowly lower your left thigh and go back to starting position.
6. Repeat the steps for 20 times.
7. After completing a set of 20 reps, rest for a bit and do another round of 20 reps.
8. Repeat the above steps on your other leg.

Tips:

- Keep your arms straight and maintain the same pressure on your right and left palms all throughout the exercise.
- Instead of just raising your leg, consider kicking your leg sideways.
- Wear a workout band a little above your knees to intensify the workout.
- Once you have mastered the basic fire hydrants, consider wearing ankle weights or workout bands.

Pictures of exercise with workout bands as shown below.

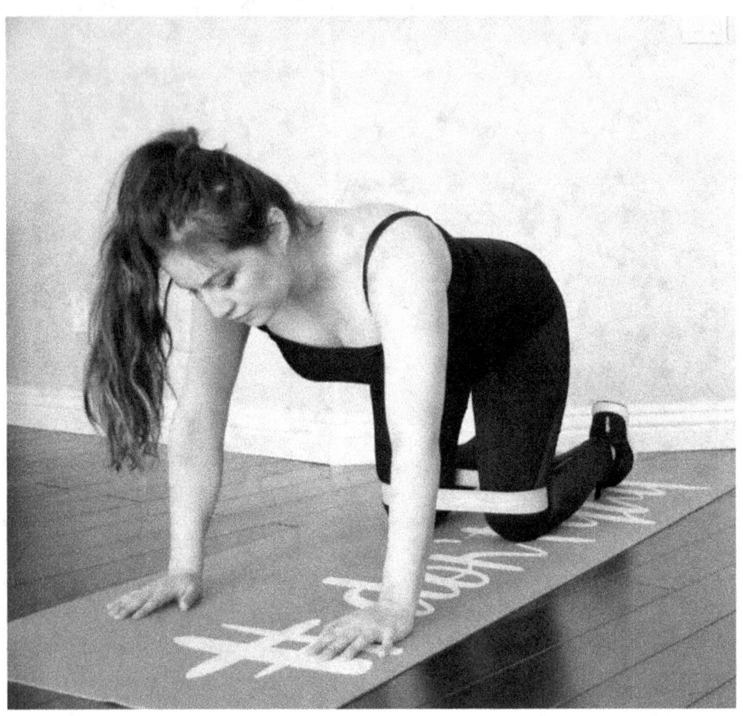

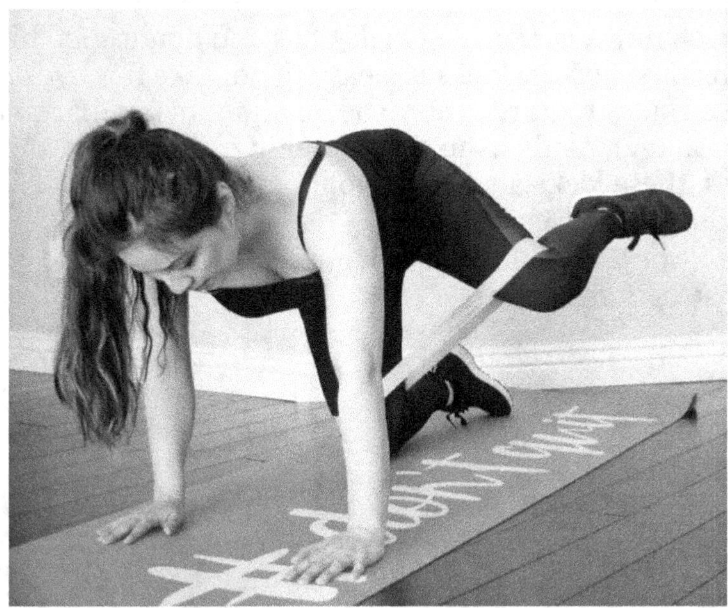

IMPORTANT:

- Skip fire hydrants if your wrists are painful.
- Don't raise your thighs beyond what you're capable of.
- If you're lower back becomes sore as your perform the exercise, tilt your pelvis up. You may not be able to raise your leg as high as before but this step can lessen or prevent the soreness.

Donkey Kicks (3 sets of 10 reps per leg)

Also known as bent-leg kickbacks and quadruped hip extensions, donkey kicks are easy to do. Like fire hydrants, donkey kicks requires you to be on all fours (similar to that of a donkey). Aside from strengthening and toning your glutes, these kicks also boost your agility and speed.

What You'll Need:

* workout mat (recommended)

Instructions:

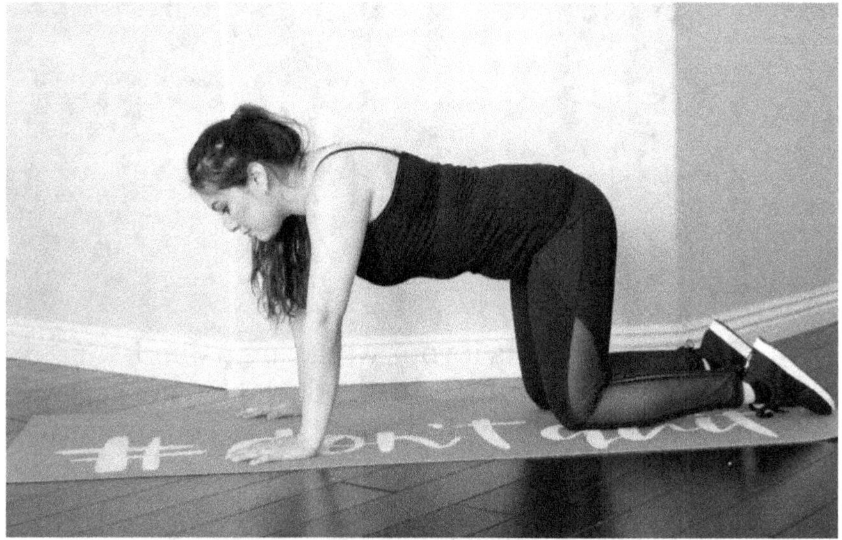

1. Get down with your palms and toes on the mat.
2. Make sure your hands are stretched out and aligned with your shoulders.
3. Bend your knees (but don't make them touch the mat) until they are aligned with your hips. Maintain a straight torso, extending from your head down to your hips, all throughout the exercise.
4. Lift your left leg but keep it bent. Your left thigh should be parallel to the floor.

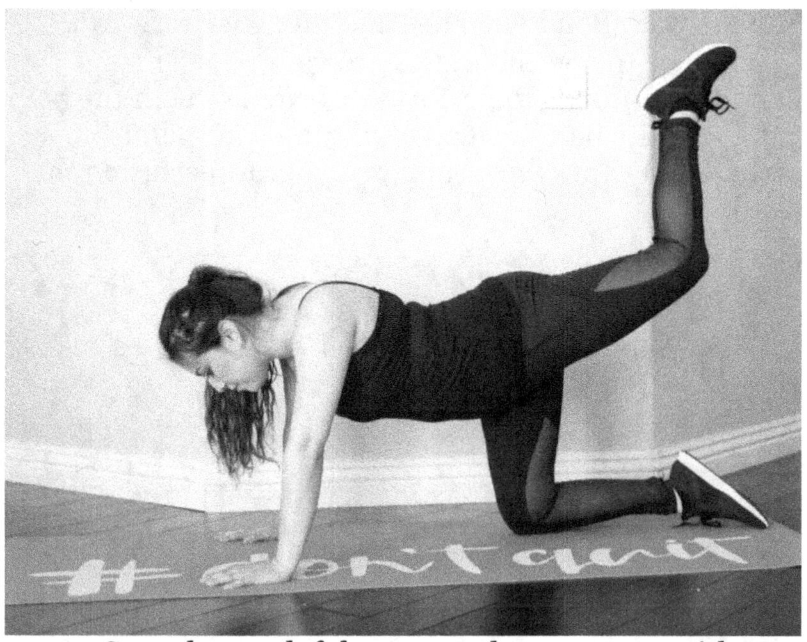

5. Stretch your left leg as much as you can without moving your upper body.
6. Lower your left leg and go back to original position.
7. Repeat the steps for 10 times.
8. After completing a set of 10 reps, rest for a bit and do two more sets of 10 reps.
9. Repeat the above steps on your other leg.

Tips:
- Perform the exercise with a workout band. There are two ways to do this:
    1. wear the workout band around your feet or legs;
    2. hold or press one end of the workout band using your hand while loop the other end around the foot you are lifting.
- You may do donkey kicks while barefoot. But if you're using a workout band, wear proper workout shoes to minimize the strain on your feet.
- If you have sore knees or wrists, you may perform donkey kicks while standing. To do this, stand facing a

wall. Extend your arms forward and put your palms
on the wall. Bend one knee and then kick forward.
- To reduce the possible strain to your sore wrists,
  another option is to perform the exercise with the help
  of a stability ball. Instead of putting your palms on a
  mat, bend your elbows and rest your forearms on the
  ball.

Side Leg Lift (2-3 sets of 15 reps per side)

Side leg lifts develop your glute and hip muscles. Another good thing about this exercise is that you can do it while watching TV. It won't tire you and make you sweat as well. You can either do it while standing up or lying on the floor. Between the two, however, doing side leg lifts while lying down is more advantageous as it engages your core.

What You'll Need:

- workout mat (recommended)

Instructions:

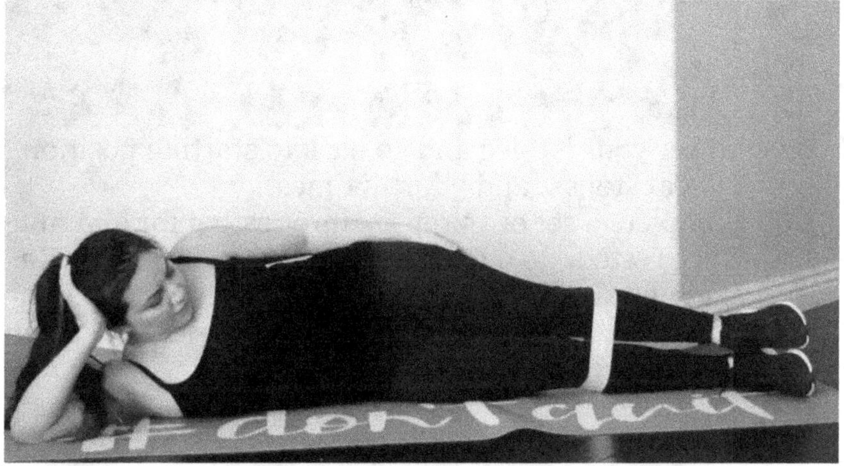

1. Lie on your right side with your legs stacked.
2. Bend your right elbow and rest your head on your right hand or forearm. Put your left hand on your hip.
3. Raise your left leg towards the ceiling (or sky if you're doing this exercise outdoors). Hold it for two to three seconds.

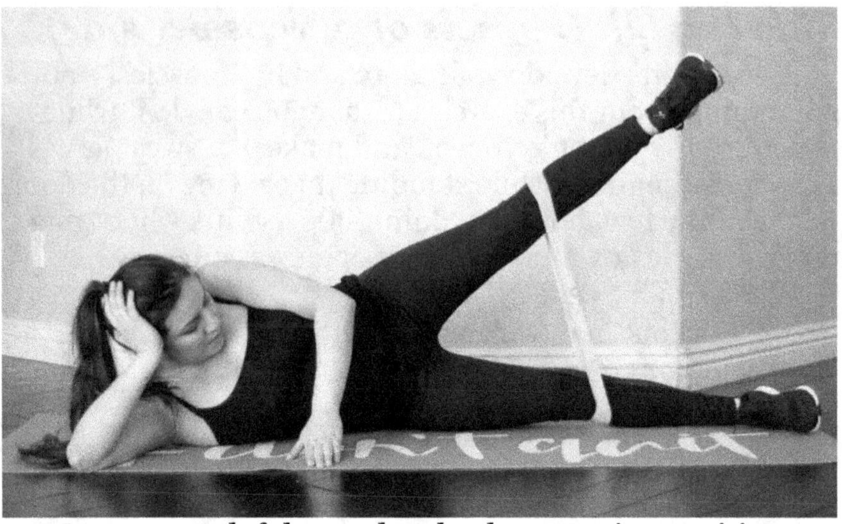

4. Lower your left leg and go back to starting position.
5. Repeat steps 2 and 3 for 15 times.
6. Complete a set of 15 reps before resting for a minute.
7. Once rested, do one or two more sets of 15 reps. Rest again for a minute.
8. Stand up and lie on your left side. Repeat the above steps on your left side.

Tips:

- To do this exercise while standing up, you may need to do it near a wall or a sturdy chair so you can have something to lean on or grab for support. But unless you have backache, do side leg lifts while lying down.
- As you perform this exercise, always keep in mind to move your hips but not your back.
- Wear a workout band below your knees to intensify the exercise.
- If you don't have a workout band, consider using ankle weights instead.

Lateral Walk (10-12 reps per side for 30-60 seconds)

The simple but highly effective lateral walk benefits your glutes and hip abductors. It strengthens the major muscles in your hips and thighs as well. Another advantage of doing this exercise is better stability and flexibility.

Instructions:

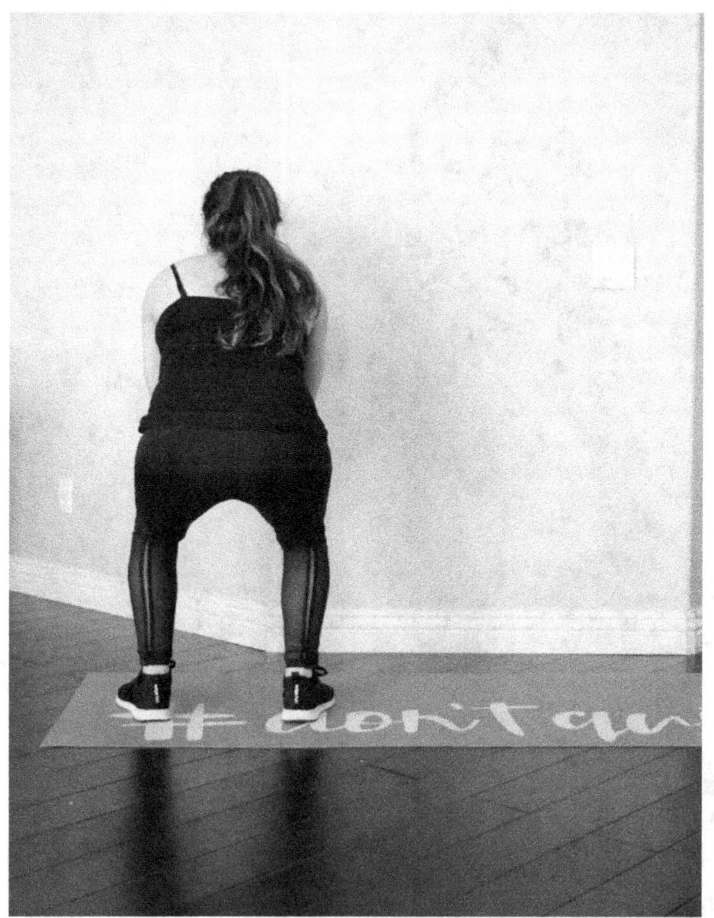

1. Put your right hand above your closed left fist. Bend your elbows, putting your hands in front of your chest.
2. Stand with your knees slight bent and feet hip-width apart.
3. Further bend your knees into squat position. Maintain this position as you complete the exercise.

4. Using your right foot, take a big step to your right.

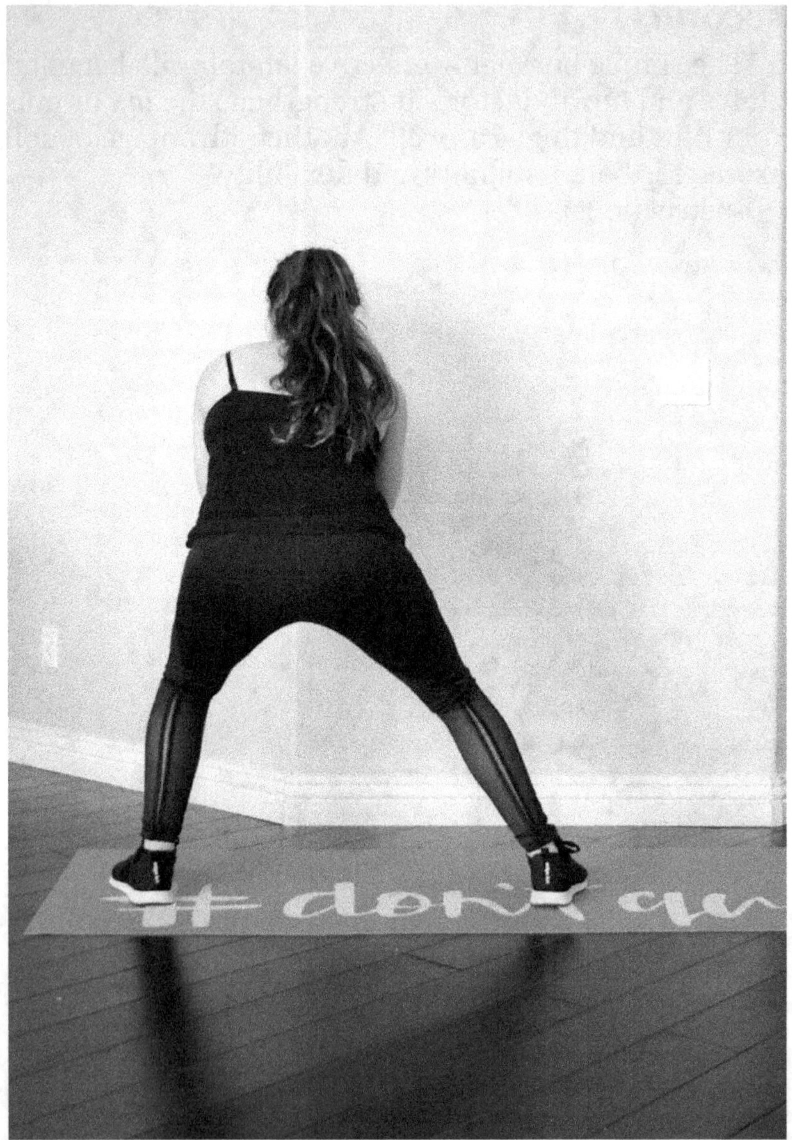

Exhale deeply as you step.

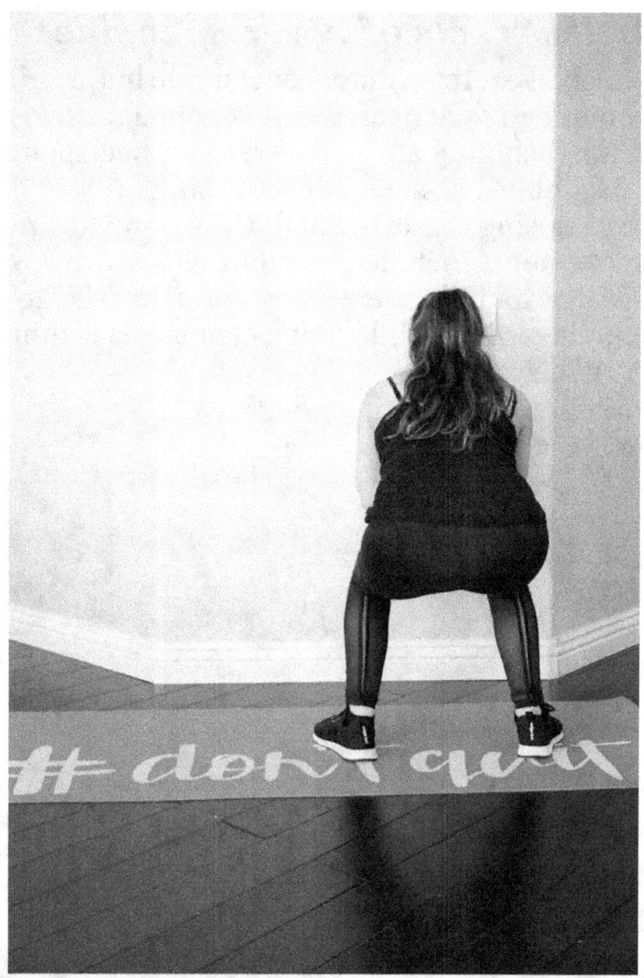

5. Using your left foot, step to your right until both feet are hip-width apart.
6. Repeat steps 4 and 5 for 10 to 12 times.
7. Rest for a bit and repeat the exercise on your left side.

Tips:
- Wear a workout band above or below your knees as you carry out this exercise. To make this more manageable, perform side leg lifts beforehand.

Clamshells (3 sets of 12 reps per side)

The clamshell exercise may seem simple but it brings notable gains such as activated glutes, toned muscles, improved hip flexibility and reduced lower back pain. The exercise was dubbed as such due to its similarity to the opening and closing of a clamshell. Unlike squats and step ups, the movements included in clamshells are awkward so it's only ideal as an indoor exercise. Though awkward, the risk of incurring injury while doing clamshells is minimal.

What You'll Need:

- workout mat (recommended)

Instructions:

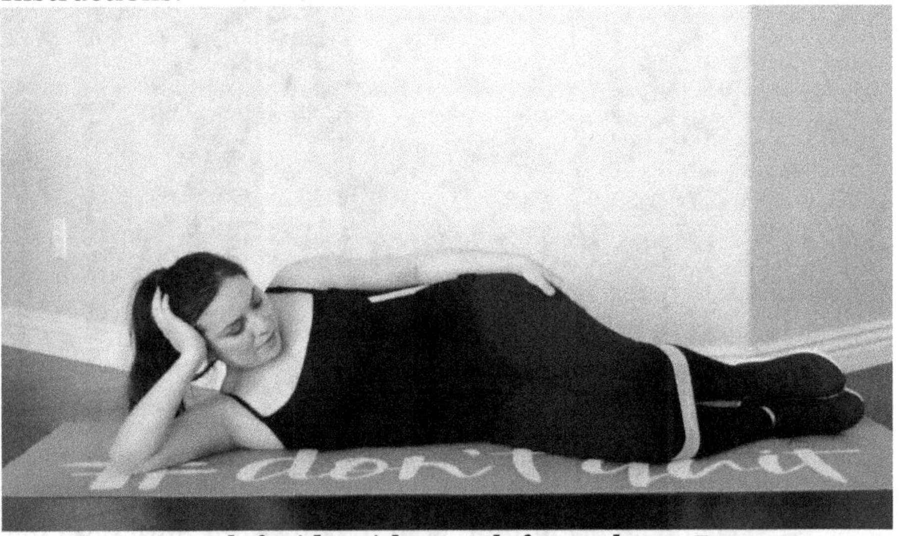

1. Lie on your left side with your left arm bent. Rest your head on your left forearm or on your palm. Keep your legs stacked and bend your knees up to an angle of 90 degrees.
2. Pull your knees towards your body. Make sure your feet are aligned with your butt.
3. Put your right hand on your hip to prevent your back from tilting.
4. Raise your right knee as high as you can but avoid moving your other knee and rotating your hip. Hold this position for a second.

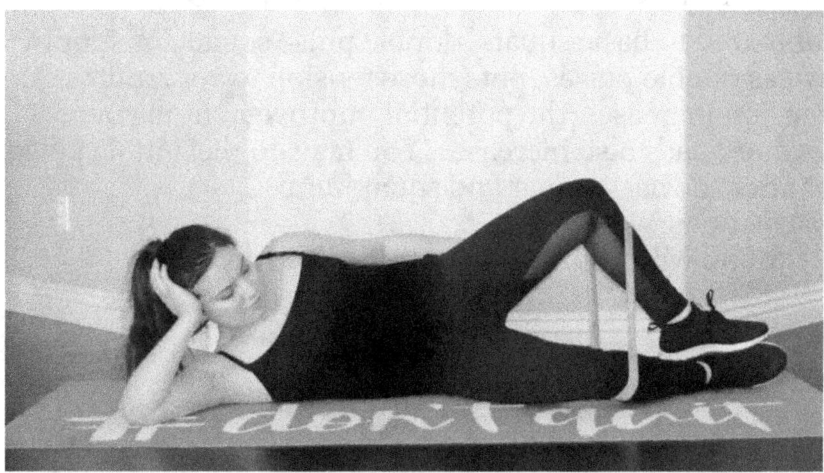

5. Tense your glutes before lowering your right knee.
6. Repeat steps 4 and 5 for 12 times.
7. After completing a set of 12 reps, rest for a bit and complete two more sets.
8. Repeat the above steps on your right side.

Tips:

- Wear a workout band around your knees as you carry out this exercise.
- Another variation of the clamshell exercise involves stability ball. Below is a guideline on how to use a stability ball while doing clamshells:
    1. Lie on your back instead of lying on your side.
    2. Put your hands behind your head for support.
    3. Bend your knees and place the stability ball in between your legs.
    4. Simultaneously lift your shoulders and legs off the floor.

Double Pulse Squat (3 sets of 10 reps)

Compared to basic squats, double pulse squats, or simply known as double pulses, puts more tension to your glutes. As the tension increases, the potential improvement in your glutes and quads also increases. You may do the double pulse squat after the basic squat and squat jump.

Instructions:

1. Stand with your feet shoulder-width apart.

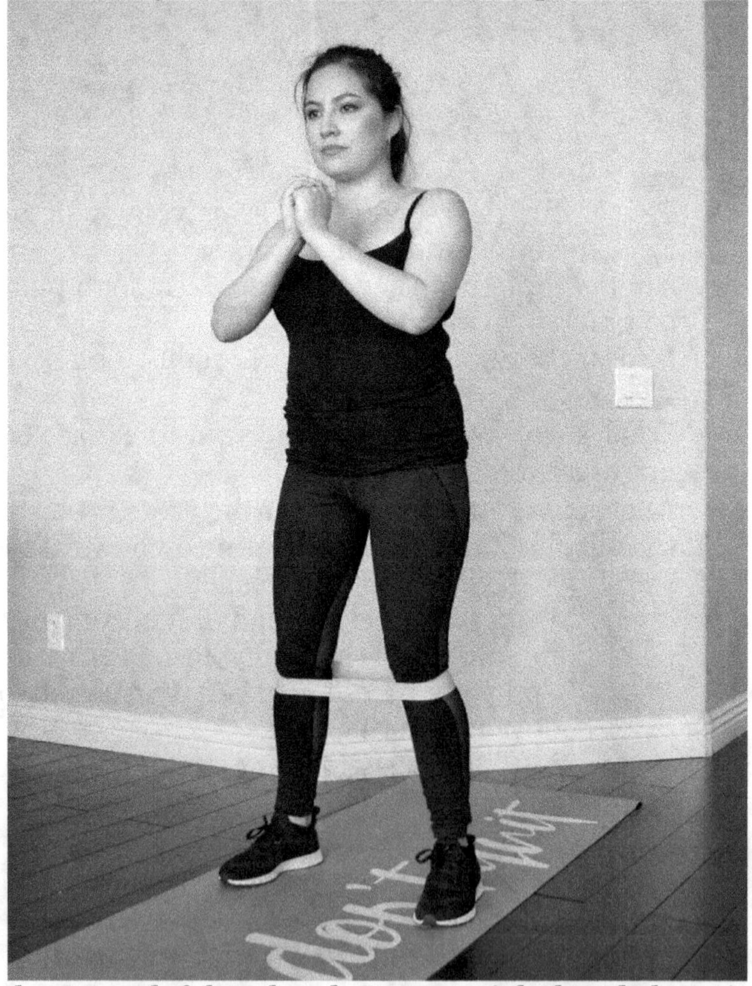

2. Close your left hand and put your right hand above it. Keep this position all throughout the exercise.
3. Tighten your core and bend your knees until they are parallel to the floor.

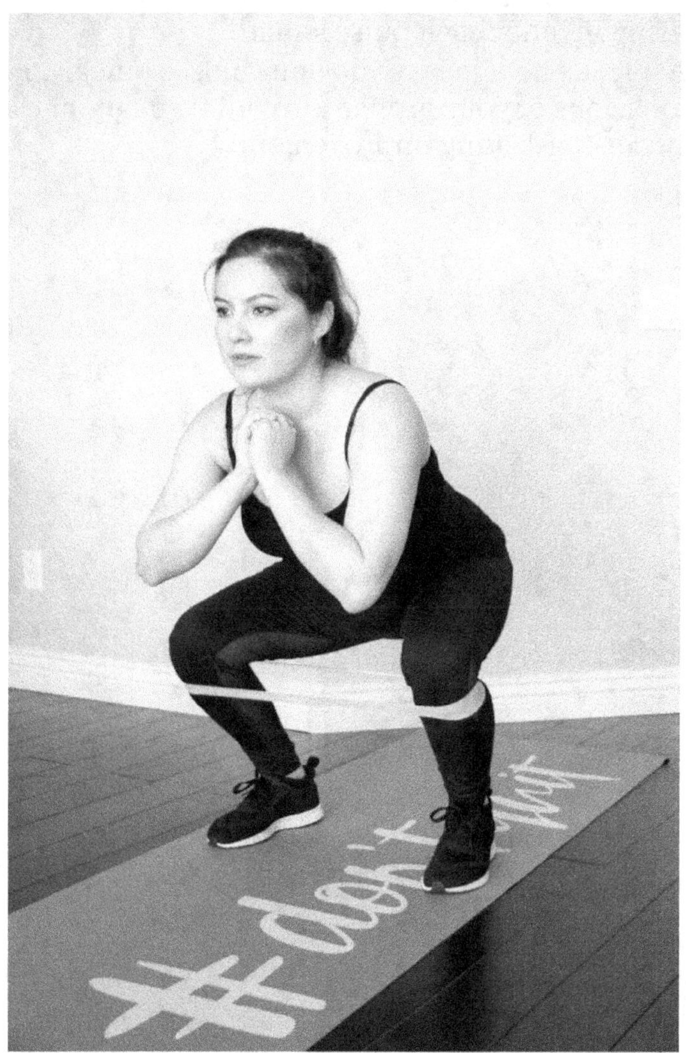

4. Rise up halfway. (Don't straighten out your knees completely.) Return to squat position. Complete step 4 within a second.
5. Repeat step 4 for 10 times.
6. Complete a set of 10 reps.
7. Rest for a minute before completing two more sets.

Tips:

*   Inhale deeply as you rise up and exhale as you squat.

- To increase the challenge, jump instead of simply rising up after each pulse squat.
- While it's beneficial to do your pulses quickly, being conscious of your proper form all throughout can offer more long-lasting improvements.

Deadlifts with Barbell or Dumbbells (3 sets of 12 reps)

The mere sight of a barbell is intimidating enough for some people. However, lifting such is one of the most beneficial exercises you can try. Aside from toning your muscles (not just glutes but also the muscles on your shoulders, arms and thighs), this activity also improves your strength and burns your extra fats. However, the risk of incurring an injury is greater with deadlifting compared to other glute exercises. Improper handling, for instance, may cause you to drop your barbell on your feet. To minimize the risk, start with a comfortable weight and be mindful of your posture all throughout the exercise.

What You'll Need:

- Barbell or dumbbells

Instructions:

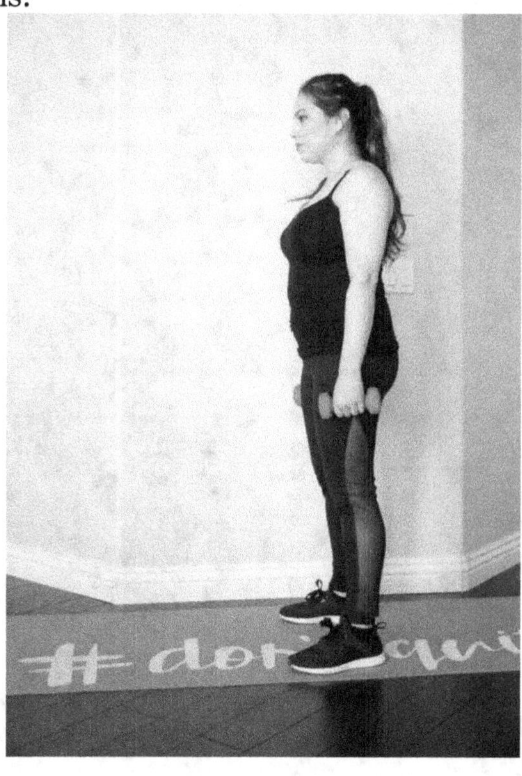

1. Stand with your feet hip-width apart in front of your barbell. Keep your back straight all throughout the exercise.
2. Bend your knees, hinge at your hips and extend your arms towards your barbell.

3. Grab the barbell with your hands a little more than shoulder-width apart.
4. Push your butt backwards until your upper body is almost parallel to the floor.
5. Keep your chest up and look forward. Press your heels to lift the barbell upwards.

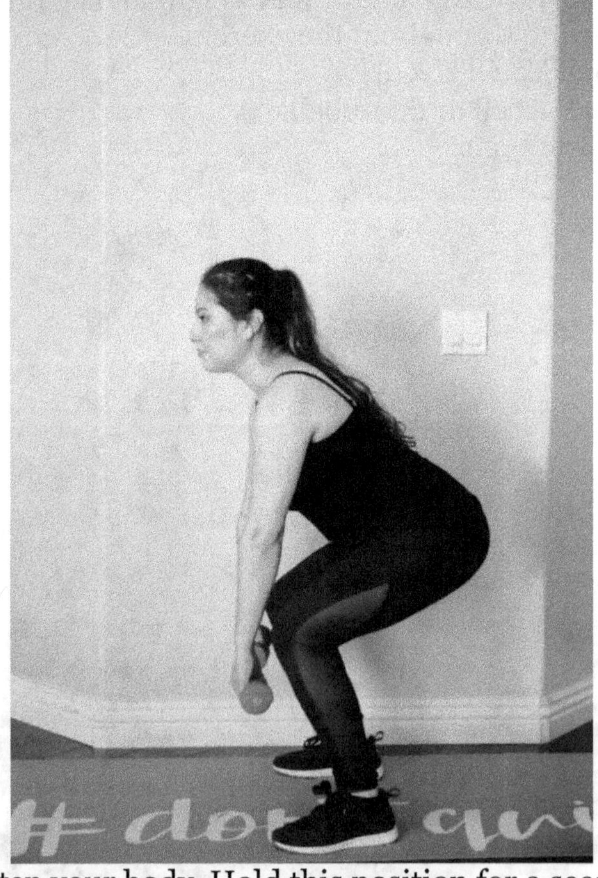

6. Straighten your body. Hold this position for a second or two.
7. Bend your hips and gently put the barbell down.

8. Repeat the steps for 12 times.

Tips:

- Don't overarch your neck while doing deadlifts.
- Always focus on good form and not on doing impressive deadlift stunts such as lifting the barbell using only one hand. With a good form, the risk of incurring injury is greatly reduced as the weight is evenly distributed.

Front Lunge (3 sets of 8 reps per leg)

Front lunge is a form of low-intensity exercise that puts emphasis on your glutes, hips, calves, quads and hamstrings. It benefits your abdominal muscles and lower back as well. As its name suggests, the front lunge is done by stepping forward. Its opposite, the reverse lunge, is done by stepping backward.

Instructions:

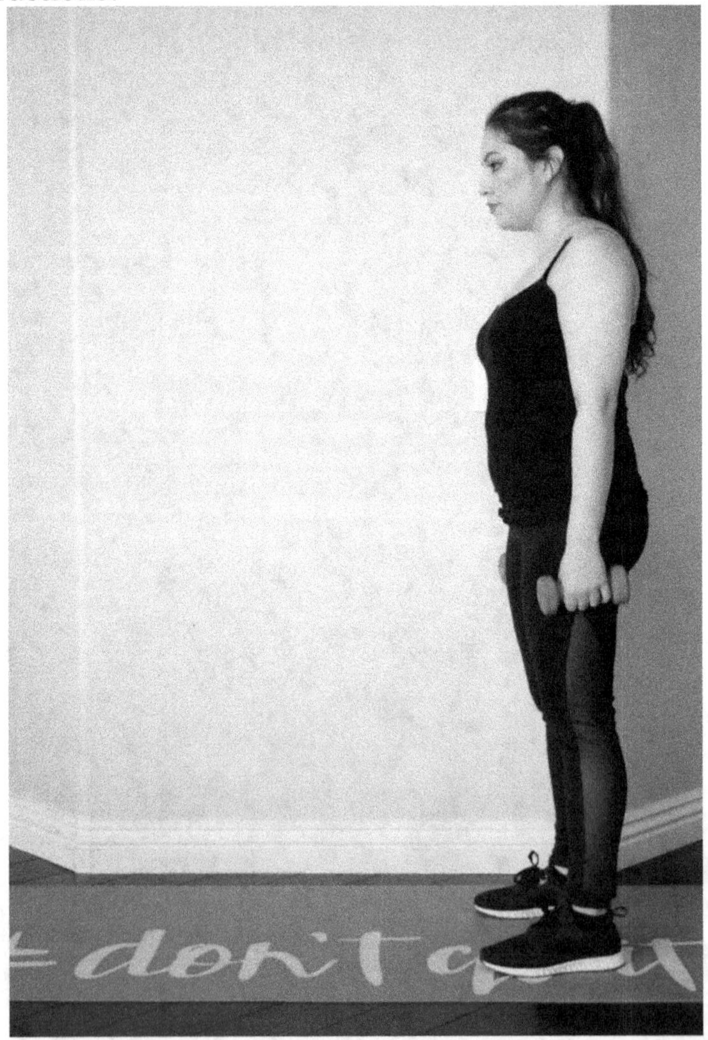

1. Stand with your hands on your hips and your feet hip-width apart.

2. Using your right leg, step forward. Transfer your weight to your right heel and make sure it hits the floor first.
3. Lower your upper body to make your right thigh parallel to the floor.

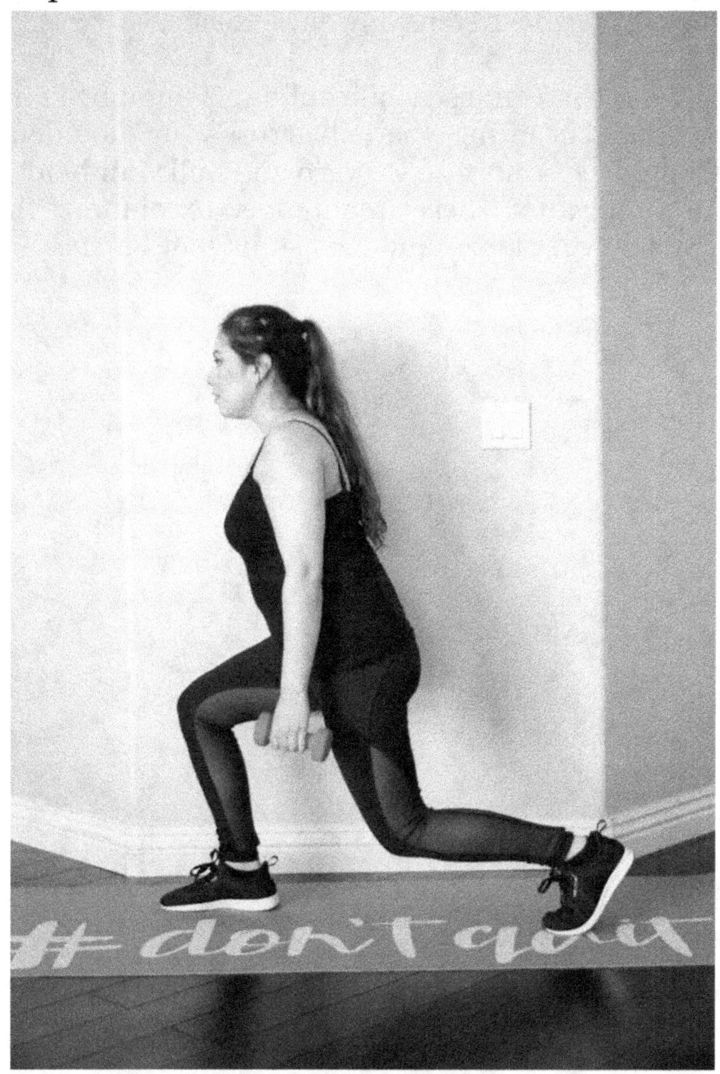

4. Keep your right shin vertical. If you can hardly do so, slightly bend your right knee but make sure it doesn't go beyond your toes.
5. Press your right heel and straighten your body, putting you back to starting position.

6. Repeat steps 2 to 5 for eight times.
7. After completing a set of eight reps on your right leg, relax for 10 to 20 seconds.
8. Complete two more sets of eight reps on your right leg.
9. Repeat the above steps on your left side.

Tips:
- Perform this exercise while holding a dumbbell on each hand or lifting a barbell across your shoulders.
- Always keep your face forward and pull your belly button inwards. These are intended to minimize the stress on your knees and to sustain your balance.

Reverse Lunge (3 sets of 8 reps per leg)

The reverse lunge is a lot similar to the front lunge, but the former has more benefits than the latter. Also dubbed as the step-back lunge, this type of exercise requires your front leg to pull away from the ground to propel yourself forward. This is basically the same movement you do when you run. So when you do reverse lunges, you're also improving your running ability. Additional benefits of reverse lunge are improved strength and flexibility, particularly on your glutes, calves and quads.

Instructions:

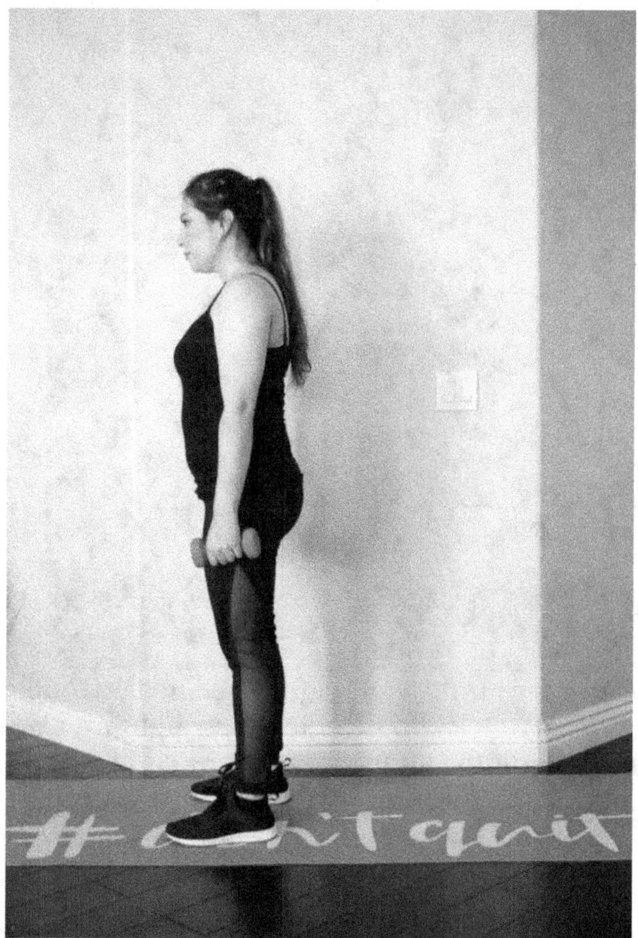

1. Stand with your hands on your hips and your feet shoulder-width apart.

2. Using your right foot, take a step backwards.

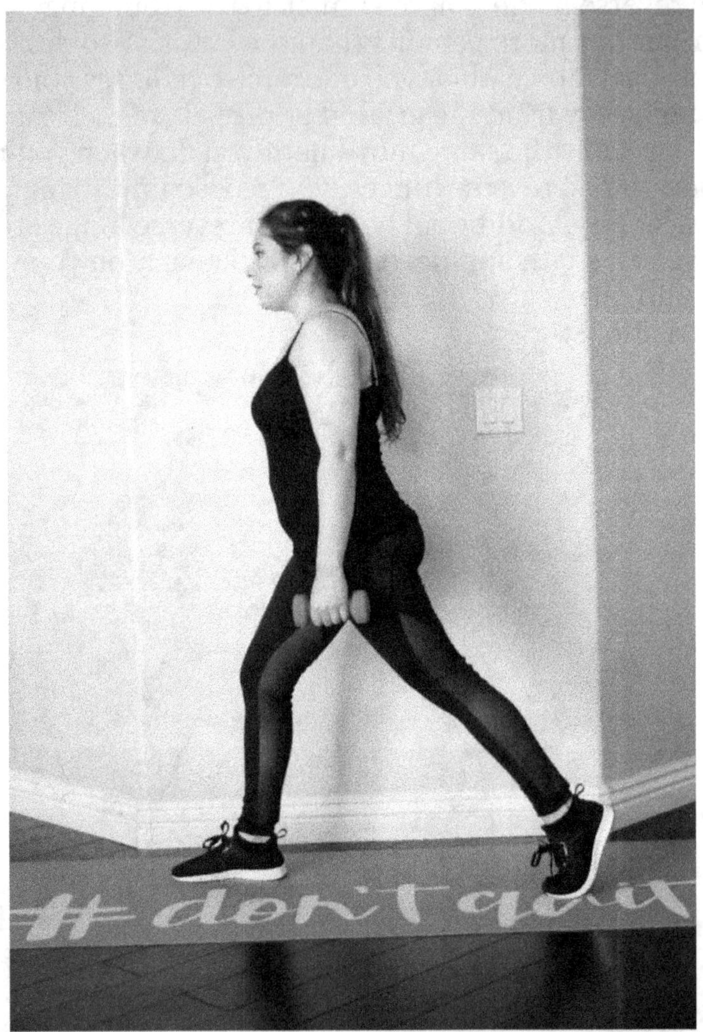

3. Bend your knees until your right knee nearly touches
    the floor. Your back should remain straight and your
    right knee should be aligned with your right foot.
    Maintain this position for three to five seconds.

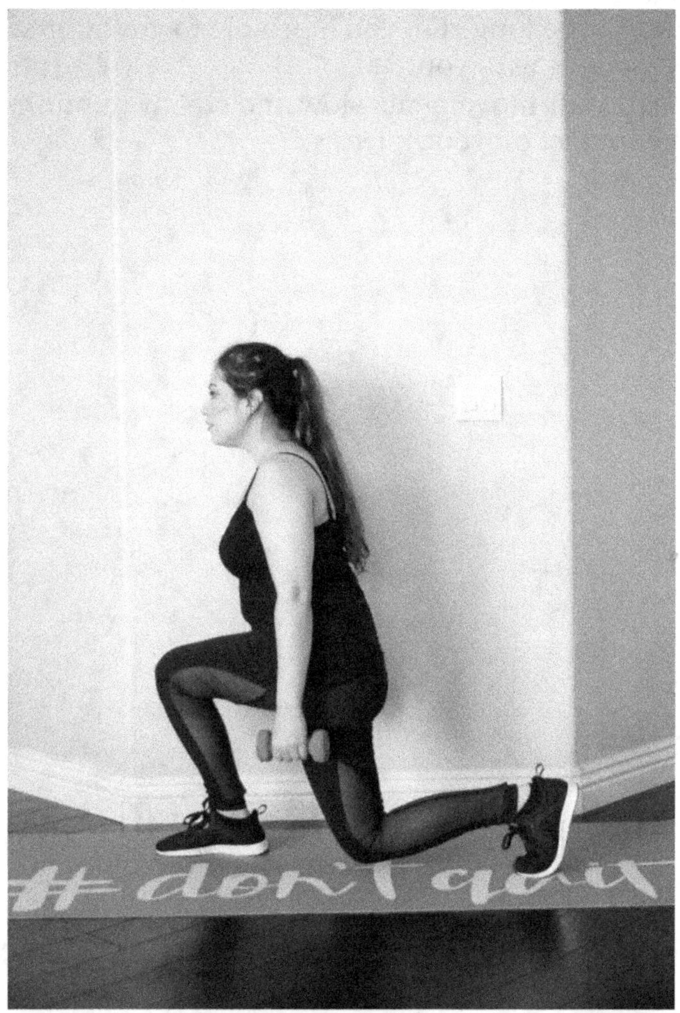

4. Put your weight on your left heel and straighten your knees.
5. Repeat steps 2 to 4 for eight times.
6. After completing a set of 8 reps, relax for 30 to 60 seconds and do two more sets of 8 reps.
7. Repeat the steps on your other leg.

Tips:

- Perform this exercise while holding a dumbbell on each hand or lifting a barbell over your shoulders.

- Avoid lunging way too low when you're just starting out. In the long run, you'll be able to go lower so just be patient with yourself.
- Keep your movements slow and steady to minimize the impact on your knees.

Perform the workouts about 2-3 times a week and see the booty take shape and increase in size! Remember consistency is key and keep at it. Performing the exercises once in awhile will not give the best results. Performing them consistency is what will allow you to start seeing changes on your body.

Additional Tips

Certain factors can make or break your attempts at glute workouts. Two of these are your diet and rest. If you want these factors to work on your favor, make sure you are getting the right quantity and quality.

Diet

Before you focus on glute exercises, you should first prioritize eliminating your body fats. Aside from working out, you should also consume a balanced diet to effectively lose fats and at the same time, provide you with the energy. This calls for cutting down your carbohydrate intake and boosting your protein intake. You should also develop beneficial eating habits such as chewing your food slowly and consuming breakfast within 90 minutes after you wake up.

Once you've shed fats, increase your protein consumption to have the energy needed to work out your glutes. Additionally, this macronutrient helps build and restore body tissues. Its tissue-restoring capability is essential as it speeds up your recovery period after each workout.

Eggs, chicken, turkey, fish, pork and dairy products are among the top sources of protein. For your snacks, you may munch on protein-rich nuts such as pistachios, almonds, cashews and walnuts. When it comes to fruit, avocados and guavas are the best choices. You may also consume bananas, apricots, peaches, kiwifruits, berries and cantaloupes every once in a while. Beans, lentils and green leafy vegetables such as kale, spinach and Brussels sprouts are other plant-based foods that can supply you with proteins.

Before you work out, prepare your own protein shake. With a durable blender, you can mix various protein-rich ingredients if you want. One simple recipe you can try is blending berries, milk and nuts. You can also make a shake out of soy milk, banana, kale and nuts. Add sweetener to suit your taste. Consider putting ice on your drink as well.

What about supplements?

The majority of supplements being advertised tend to target weight loss and memory enhancement. These days, though, there are also supplements made for improving butt size. Nevertheless, these are too few. Therefore, the studies backing their efficiency are rare, if not inexistent.

Protein supplements may be worth considering if you're not too keen on lengthy meal preparations. However, you shouldn't depend on such products for your entire protein needs. They may be made to provide you with more of the said macronutrient but they may also come with side effects. Plus, you can't fully control the distribution of proteins in your body. The extra proteins you may gain from supplements may end up developing muscles in other parts of your body instead of your butt.

Rest

You're not supposed to perform the glute exercises every day to achieve your dream booty size sooner. In fact, it's not advisable to do so as daily squatting, for instance, can do more damage than good. Don't even try to allot a workout session in the morning and another one in the afternoon. Allow your muscles to recover first because if you don't, they'll be more prone to inflammation and injury. So make sure you have a rest day included in every week of glute workouts.

Other Lifestyle Changes

Relaxation is a key component of a healthy lifestyle although it's often overshadowed by exercise and diet. Feeling relaxed most of the time improves your concentration. This is essential when you are working in the office, driving home or exercising. But with so many stressors around, being at ease seems impossible.

It's hard to focus on your workout when you're stressed. Moreover, no matter how hard you try to follow a workout and diet plan, being stressed will prevent your body from forming muscles. So as you enhance your physique, learn to work on your stressors as well. To relieve your stress, indulge yourself in massages and bond with your loved ones. One bonding activity you can try is working out.

It also pays to set a schedule for specific tasks at home. This should include your time for eating, preparing meals, sleeping, waking up and working out. Following a set schedule may help discourage you from unproductive habits such as watching TV and browsing your social media feeds for an hour.

Results may vary

Many people claim about enhancing their butt size by doing so-called 30-day challenges. Don't be deceived by their claims, though. Unless you've been a fitness buff for quite a long time, ditching your old habits and forming new, positive ones will take a lot of time. When you're feeling discouraged about the lack of significant results on your bum, weigh on the other benefits of carrying out glute exercises.

As long as you are consistent with the workouts provided, you will definitely see results! There may be times where you feel like there has not been any changes but try to push through and keep going. As I have mentioned before, a great way to see noticeable results is before starting the workouts, take a picture of your body, maybe from the side view of the booty as an example. After doing these workouts consistently for about a month, take another photo. You should definitely notice a difference between the pictures and use that as motivation to continue!

Another very important tip is to not compare yourself to the fitness models you may see on social media, Instagram, etc. It is easy to start comparing your own body to theirs but try not to. Be reasonable with your expectations and set small goals. It is going to take time to reach your goals to increase your booty size but consistency is key! Stay consistent and you WILL see results!

Conclusion

Thanks again for downloading this book!

I hope that this book was able to provide the necessary information and inspiration you need to improve your butt size. Hopefully, with the knowledge you get from this book, you also gain the confidence and discipline to carry out the exercises included herein. Most importantly, I wish that this encouraged you to make healthier lifestyle choices, not just for the enhancement of your bum, but for your overall wellness.

The next step is to fully commit to a healthy lifestyle. That way, maintaining your plump bum is easier. While they may eventually sag due to old age, the most important thing is you're able to maximize their use and enjoy their appeal for a long time.

Good luck!